Essentials of the Spine

Essentials of the Spine

Editors

James N. Weinstein, D.O.
Director, Spine Diagnostic and Treatment Center
Department of Orthopaedic Surgery
The University of Iowa Hospitals and Clinics
Iowa City, Iowa

Björn L. Rydevik, M.D., Ph.D.
Associate Professor of Orthopaedic Surgery
Department of Orthopaedics
Sahlgren University Hospital
Gothenburg, Sweden

Volker K.H. Sonntag, M.D., F.A.C.S.
Vice Chairman, Barrow Neurological Institute
Chairman, Spine Section
Barrow Neurological Institute
Phoenix, Arizona; and
Clinical Professor of Neurosurgery
Division of Neurological Surgery
University of Arizona
Tucson, Arizona

Raven Press ✹ New York

Raven Press, Ltd., 1185 Avenue of the Americas, New York, New York 10036

Made in the United States of America

Library of Congress Cataloging-in-Publication Data

Essentials of the Spine / James N. Weinstein, Björn L. Rydevik, Volker K.H.
   Sonntag, editors.
         p.   cm.
      Includes bibliographical references and index.
      ISBN 0-7817-0251-8
      1. Spine—Diseases.   2. Spine—Abnormalities.   3. Spine—Wounds
   and injuries.   I. Weinstein, James N.   II. Rydevik, Björn L.
   III. Sonntag, Volker K.H.
      [DNLM: 1. Spinal Diseases—diagnosis.   2. Spinal Diseases—therapy.
   3. Spinal Diseases—physiopathology.   WE 725 E78 1995]
   RD533.E87   1995
   616.7'3—dc20
   DNLM/DLC
   for Library of Congress   94-38406
                                                                    CIP

9 8 7 6 5 4 3 2 1

Contents

Contributing Authors

Gunnar B.J. Andersson, M.D., Ph.D. *Professor and Acting Chairman, Department of Orthopedic Surgery, Rush-Presbyterian-St. Luke's Medical Center, 1653 West Congress Parkway, Chicago, Illinois 60612, USA*

Scott D. Boden, M.D. *Assistant Professor of Orthopaedic Surgery, Department of Orthopaedic Surgery, Emory University School of Medicine, The Emory Spine Center, 2165 North Decatur Road, Decatur, Georgia 30033, USA*

Richard A. Deyo, M.D., M.P.H. *Professor of Medicine and Health Services, Departments of Medicine and Health Services, University of Washington, 3747 15th Avenue NE, Seattle, Washington 98105, USA*

Steven R. Garfin, M.D. *Professor, Department of Orthopaedics, University of California at San Diego, 200 West Arbor Drive, San Diego, California 92103-8894, USA*

Edward N. Hanley, Jr., M.D. *Chairman, Department of Orthopaedic Surgery, Carolinas Medical Center, 1000 Blythe Boulevard, Suite 503, Charlotte, North Carolina 28203, USA*

Mitsuo Hasue, M.D. *Department of Orthopedic Surgery, Japanese Red Cross Medical Center, Tokyo, Japan*

Harry N. Herkowitz, M.D. *Chairman, Department of Orthopaedic Surgery, William Beaumont Hospital, Medical Office Building, 3535 West Thirteen Mile Road, Suite 604, Royal Oak, Michigan 48073-6705, USA*

Richard J. Herzog, M.D. *Associate Professor of Radiology, Department of Radiology, Hospital of the University of Pennsylvania, 3400 Spruce Street, Philadelphia, Pennsylvania 19104, USA*

Jeffrey D. Klein, M.D. *Attending Orthopaedic Surgeon, Department of Orthopaedic Surgery, Hospital for Joint Diseases Orthopaedic Institute, 301 East 17th Street, New York, New York 10003, USA*

Kjell Olmarker, M.D., Ph.D. *Associate Research Professor, Department of Orthopaedics, Sahlgren University Hospital, S-413 45 Gothenburg, Sweden*

Richard W. Porter, M.D., F.R.C.S., F.R.C.S.E. *Professor of Orthopaedic Surgery, Department of Orthopaedic Surgery, Aberdeen University, Foresterhill, AB9 2ZD Aberdeen, United Kingdom*

Björn L. Rydevik, M.D., Ph.D.   *Associate Professor of Orthopaedic Surgery, Department of Orthopaedics, Sahlgren University Hospital, S-413 45 Gothenburg, Sweden*

Volker K.H. Sonntag, M.D., F.A.C.S.   *Vice Chairman, Barrow Neurological Institute, Chairman, Spine Section, Barrow Neurological Institute, 350 West Thomas Road, Phoenix, Arizona 85013-4496, USA; and Clinical Professor of Neurosurgery, Division of Neurological Surgery, University of Arizona, Tucson, Arizona 85724, USA*

James N. Weinstein, D.O.   *Director, Spine Diagnostic and Treatment Center, Department of Orthopaedic Surgery, The University of Iowa Hospitals and Clinics, 200 Hawkins Drive, Iowa City, Iowa 52242, USA*

Stuart L. Weinstein, M.D.   *Ignacio V. Ponseti Professor of Orthopaedic Surgery, Department of Orthopaedic Surgery, University of Iowa Hospitals, 1012 Carver Pavilion, Iowa City, Iowa 52242, USA*

Sam W. Wiesel, M.D.   *Professor and Chairman, Department of Orthopaedic Surgery, Georgetown University Hospital, 3800 Reservoir Road NW, Washington, DC 20007, USA*

Preface

Our motivation for developing *Essentials of the Spine* originated from our teaching experiences at the University of Iowa Hospitals and Clinics, the Sahlgren University Hospital in Gothenburg, Sweden, and the Barrow Neurological Institute in Phoenix, Arizona. Our students have repeatedly suggested that their learning would be enhanced by a book that would serve as an aid during the clinical rotation and as a reference resource once the rotation was completed.

All of the contributors to the book have delivered lectures and conducted seminars for groups ranging from residents and physicians of the various spine societies to media representatives, biomechanical engineers, neurophysiologists, internists, and other investigators whose primary interest is in the basic science and clinical study of the spine. The universal concerns expressed by all of these diverse groups have been how to evaluate the literature regarding the spine, and how to determine its value to their particular areas of interest. We believe these concerns are both important and timely. The importance of gaining such insights is borne out by the fact that much of continuing medical education is derived from the current literature. The timeliness is reflected in the large quantity of information from the literature that is now disseminated daily to the general public by the media.

Careful application of clinical principles and methods requires the development of a particular way of thinking, which we have incorporated into this primer. Our major objective is to enable the readers, be they medical or surgical residents, family physicians, chiropractors, internists, or researchers to interpret and apply these basic principles to their own particular needs. We hope this book will facilitate collaboration among the various specialties so that collectively we may better understand the methods employed in the pursuit of more valid clinical assessments. For the smaller subgroup of readers who will pursue a career in the study of the spine, we hope this book will provide a useful bridge to more advanced concepts and textbooks.

To improve our diagnostic and treatment abilities, physicians must use the available tools more precisely and become cognizant of their limitations. The physical examination and history remain the basis for all spine diagnosis. The results of this initial examination should be the guide to further decisions and testing. To perform these tests in a logical sequence, physicians must be aware of the accuracy of these tests and how they relate to patient treatment and outcomes. We have particularly tried to present the principles and methods related to the most appropriate clinical diagnosis and treatment algorithms in as clear and concise a manner as possible.

Examples from our own practices are used to illustrate current diagnostic and therapeutic tools of importance.

We have attempted to achieve a balanced perspective between an exposition of clinical and basic science as they relate to dealing with patients presenting with various spinal maladies. The combined experience of our outstanding authors and their understanding and application of clinical methodologies from various viewpoints will provide the reader with a greater understanding of the spine and its associated disorders.

Anyone who treats or strives to understand the spine—from the resident to the spine specialist—needs to continually refresh and update knowledge of diagnosis and treatment. *Essentials of the Spine* is designed to meet that need.

James N. Weinstein
Björn L. Rydevik
Volker K.H. Sonntag

Essentials of the Spine

1

Epidemiology

Gunnar B. J. Andersson

Department of Orthopedic Surgery, Rush-Presbyterian-St. Luke's Medical Center, Chicago, Illinois 60612, USA

Key Points

- The 1-yr prevalence of back pain is 30% to 60%.

- About 2% of the U.S. work force has a work-related back injury each year; the incidence is similar in other industrialized countries.

- Back pain is the most common cause of activity limitation in persons less than 45 years of age.

- The natural history of back pain is very favorable; most episodes resolve in 10 to 30 days.

- Two percent to 7% of people develop chronic back pain, and 1% to 3% require surgery.

Epidemiology is the study of occurrence rates of diseases and of the determinants of those occurrences. The epidemiology of low back pain is important for at least three reasons. If we know the size and distribution of the back problem, we can predict the demand on medical services and direct our resources appropriately. Determination of the natural history of back problems makes it possible to inform patients accurately and also to determine whether treatment results in changes in the natural history. Studies of associations between low back pain and individual, work-related, and other factors allow hypothesis testing and the development of new hypotheses that can be tested experimentally.

DEFINITIONS

The *prevalence* of back pain or sciatica is defined as the number of people in a given population who have those complaints at a particular time. Prevalence is further defined by the time period. The *point prevalence* of back pain means back pain at the time the question is asked, whereas, for example, a 1-mo prevalence means back pain occurring during the past month. Prevalence can be determined by a single survey and is, therefore, an inexpensive and practical measure. *Incidence,* on the other hand, is a measure of the number of people without back pain and sciatica who will develop such pain over a defined period. The determination of incidence requires following a population over time and, therefore, is a more expensive and time-consuming effort.

DIFFICULTIES

Because there is a lack of general agreement on diagnosis and classification, because of the difficulty in studying pain epidemiologically, and because there are often no objective signs of back pain, its epidemiology is at best approximate. Some investigators have in fact suggested that epidemiologic research should be done only on conditions such as sciatica or disc herniation where the definitions are more stable. This limits the usefulness of studies to those conditions, however, and they include only a small part of all back complaints. Another problem in back epidemiology is that the sources of information about prevalence and incidence are of variable quality. The best sources from a quality perspective, such as insurance and hospital data, are not readily available and cover only a part of the problem. For example, only a few of all workers with back pain will, in fact, file a claim, and less than 1% of patients

with back pain require surgery. Other data sources are questionnaires and interviews, which have questionable validity and reliability. The answers depend on the formulation of the questions, and misinterpretations occur. The intermittent nature of back symptoms make cross-section prevalence studies difficult, and retrospective studies have problems in terms of recall.

In studies of relationships between back pain and occupational risk factors, there is also the problem of measuring exposure. Further, the so-called *healthy worker effect* introduces a bias because it allows healthy workers to stay in the same occupation while workers with back pain may have to leave their job and move on to a less demanding one. This will obviously influence the job-specific prevalence. Compensation and socioeconomic issues add to the problem, particularly when workers' compensation data are used. Also, epidemiologic data do not prove causality and, therefore, all conclusions must be interpreted with caution and related to experimental findings.

THE PREVALENCE OF BACK PAIN, INCLUDING SCIATICA

Two U.S. national surveys performed in the 1970s included questions about back pain. Those were the National Health and Nutrition Examination Survey (NHANES I) performed in 1970–74 and NHANES II performed in 1976– 80. In NHANES I, the prevalence of self-reported symptoms was 17%, while 1% were estimated as having had a disc disorder. This is a fairly low figure compared to other prevalence studies, which is explained by the fact that back pain was defined as having lasted for at least 2 wk. In NHANES II, the cumulative lifetime prevalence (back pain at some time in life) of 2 wk of back pain was 13.8%, while 1.6% reported that they had ongoing or previous sciatica. In NHANES II, the peak prevalence of back pain occurred in the 55–64 year age group, while the highest prevalence of sciatica occurred in the 45–54 year age interval (Fig. 1). This illustrates the difference between back pain and sciatica in terms of age-related prevalence.

More recent data from national health interview surveys (1985–88) show that back disorders on average resulted in 175 million lost workdays each year. The most common diagnosis for these patients was back sprain, which, each year, resulted in the hospitalization of as many as 100,000 patients. For sciatica and so-called disc disorders, the same studies revealed that, annually, 4.1 million people were affected. Back pain is the most frequent cause of activity limitation among people below age 45 and is the second most common cause for physician visits among all chronic disorders. Other data sources such as the National Hospital Discharge Data (1988) show that intervertebral disc disorders are at the top of musculoskeletal conditions leading to over 400,000 hospitalization episodes per year. The number of operations for spinal conditions has increased in the United States during the 1980s. In 1987, there were 38 laminectomies per 100,000 inhabitants, while the number of discectomies was 103 and the number of lumbar fusions 15. These numbers have increased further in the 1990s, and it is now estimated that well over 300,000 back operations are performed annually in the United States.

Data from the United Kingdom is quite similar to those from the United States Thus, in 1988–89, low back pain was the single largest cause of sick leave, accounting for 12.5% of all sick days. In 1992–93 there were 81 million sick days with a back diagnosis, 7 million visits to general practitioners for back pain, and 33,000 work-related injuries. Swedish sickness absence

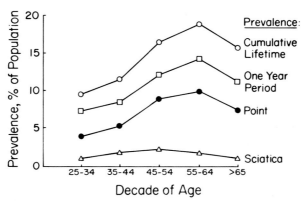

FIG. 1. Prevalence of back pain and sciatica in the United States lasting for at least 2 wk. (Adapted from Deyo and Tsui-Wu (1987), with permission.)

data reveal that back pain was responsible for 13.5% of all sickness absence days in 1987, or a total of 14.8 million lost work days. Canadian, German, Dutch, and Finnish statistics also attest to the international similarities in back pain prevalence.

Although the data on prevalence compares well between countries, there are differences in the rates of back surgery. Back surgery rates are much higher in the United States than elsewhere. A comparison among 13 different countries reveals that the back surgery rate in the United States is at least 40% higher than that in any of the other countries and is more than five times higher than those of Scotland and England. For discectomies, the number of people operated on in Great Britain has been estimated at 100/million/year, compared to Sweden 200/million/year, Finland 350/million/year, and the United States 1,310/million/year. This big difference in procedures between countries is probably not a reflection of the prevalence of disease but, rather, of differences in socioeconomic, legal, and health care systems.

Cross-sectional studies of different populations show remarkably similar prevalence rates among countries and regions within the same country. The cumulative lifetime prevalence in the cross-sectional studies is much higher than in the previously discussed NHANES studies because a 2-wk symptom period was usually not required. Thus, these studies indicate that 60% to 80% of people have low back pain at some time in life. Typically, the peak prevalence increases with increasing age. However, this age-related increase seems to be more pronounced in women than

in men, perhaps reflecting the problem of osteoporosis (Fig. 2). Point prevalence rates vary from 12% to 35%, with multiple studies reporting prevalence rates around 30%. In other words, on any given day, every third to fourth adult person will have a back problem.

Low back pain is not confined to adults only, however. About one third of all

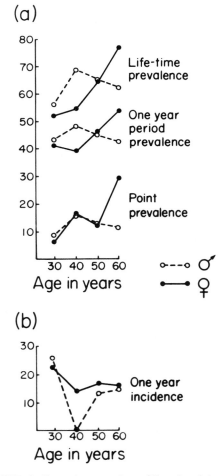

FIG. 2. Prevalence rates of "low back trouble" by age and sex. (Adapted from Biering-Sorensen (1982), with permission.)

school children have back pain at some time, and about 15% of all children have disabling pain or have received medical care for back pain.

THE PREVALENCE
OF NECK PAIN

There is little general information on how commonly neck pain occurs, and not infrequently neck pain is combined with shoulder disorders in those statistics. Cross-sectional studies, primarily from Scandinavia, report 1-yr prevalence rates of 12% to 18%.

THE PREVALENCE
OF OCCUPATIONAL
LOW BACK PAIN

Back pain is a large problem for industry. Most information about occupational back injuries comes from disability claims. Disability is a more severe expression of back pain than is just a simple report of having pain. This is reflected in the fact that the 1-yr incidence of back symptoms ranges between some 30% and 60% in working populations, while only 2% to 5% file injury claims or seek medical care. In the United States, it is estimated that about 2% of the working population have a compensable back injury each year, with an annual number of injuries of about 500,000. The U.S. data are consistent with data from Canada with respect to the 1-yr incidence and are also consistent with data from the United Kingdom and Scandinavia. About 90% of all work-related injuries are caused by manual material handling, and most are labeled as back sprains or strains. Although there are large local variations in sprain and strain rates, the average annually reported incidence per 100 workers ranges from 0.75 to 4.5. Prevalence rates are generally higher for workers in physically demanding jobs. This reflects not only the risk but also the difficulty of performing heavy jobs with a painful low back. Indeed, back pain is very frequent in physically light jobs as well and, therefore, a change in work environment alone cannot be expected to solve the back injury problem completely.

THE PREVALENCE
OF OCCUPATIONAL NECK PAIN

The frequency of neck pain in different industrial populations is quite high, approaching and sometimes surpassing that of low back pain. The symptoms seem to be less severe, however, and are diffuse, often combined with shoulder and arm discomfort or pain. Physically demanding work, particularly in the meat industry, has a high prevalence rate, as have jobs where there are requirements to maintain a certain head position or to bend or turn the neck frequently or for prolonged periods. Thus, prevalence rates are high among dentists, data entry operators, and certain assembly line workers, with complaints of daily symptoms from 4% to 20%.

OCCUPATIONAL FACTORS
IN LOW BACK PAIN

The seven most frequently discussed occupational factors are listed in Table 1. Six of those factors are physical work factors and have been experimentally associated with the development of injuries to different spinal tissues. The seventh,

TABLE 1. *Occupational factors associated with an increased risk of low back pain*

Heavy physical work
Frequent bending and twisting
Lifting, pushing, and pulling
Repetitive work
Static work postures
Vibrations
Psychologic and psychosocial factors

which is the psychologic and psychosocial factor, is probably more related to disability than to a specific injury.

Almost all existing information indicates that physically heavy work increases the risk of back pain, sciatica, and disc herniation. This is true both for national statistics and for cross-sectional studies of various populations. It is also true for different countries and different types of physically heavy work environments. Yet it is still unclear whether physical loading is an etiologic factor or primarily acts to exacerbate symptoms from already existing conditions. Lifting is often part of physically heavy work and is a well-known triggering event for back pain. Some studies show that back pain in workers doing heavy manual lifting is as much as eight times more common than in those doing lighter physical work. Other studies show that compensable back injuries are up to three times more common among workers who do excessive manual handling and that disc herniations occur up to six times as often in people who do frequent lifting, particularly in conjunction with bending and twisting of the back. Frequent bending and twisting, as such, also seems to increase the risk of back pain, as does repetitive work. It is generally believed

that the reason for the increased risk in physically demanding jobs has to do with the influence of mechanical loading on the lower back which, particularly if loading is repetitive, can cause significant injury to different spinal tissues. The exposures needed to create a back problem are still unknown, and there are no practical methods available to measure exposure over time.

Work for long periods in unchanged posture, such as long-term sitting, can result in muscular fatigue and injury and is another known factor associated with an increased risk of back pain. Sitting may be a contributing factor to why drivers of motor vehicles have an increased risk of back pain. It is believed, however, that this is also related to the whole-body vibration to which the drivers are exposed. Studies show that not only the risk of back pain but also the risk of disc herniation is increased in professional motor vehicle drivers.

As stated above, the psychologic and psychosocial work factors are probably most important in terms of their influence on back disability. Prospective studies show that these factors are strong predictors of the risk of future back injury reports and sickness absences. Workplace changes to reduce the risk of back injuries, therefore, should involve the psychologic work environment as well.

INDIVIDUAL FACTORS IN LOW BACK PAIN

Eight individual factors have been particularly discussed in the context of low back pain (Table 2). Of those eight, only age and sex seem to be associated with

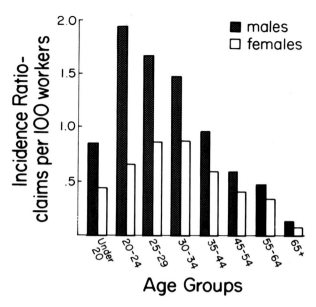

FIG. 3. Incidence ratio (claims per 100 workers and year) of compensation claims in 26 U.S. states due to sprains/strains of the back. (Adapted from Klein et al. (1984), with permission.)

TABLE 2. *Individual factors often discussed as potential risk factors in low back pain*

Factor	Importance
Age	Certain
Sex	Probable (age-dependent)
Posture	Low (severe only)
Anthropometry	Low (extremes only)
Muscle strength	Low (work-related)
Physical fitness	Low (work-related)
Spine mobility	Low
Smoking	Probable

increased risk. As stated previously, back pain often occurs for the first time early in life. The highest prevalence rates for back pain occur in the 35–55 year age range for men, whereas women have somewhat higher prevalence rates even later in life (Fig. 2). The highest risk for low back disability caused by work-related injuries, however, is in men who are in their twenties (Fig. 3). Operations for disc herniations occur most frequently in back patients who are in the early forties and are about twice as common in men as in women (Fig. 4). This is in spite of the fact that the prevalence rates for back pain for women and men are quite similar.

Postural deformities, such as scoliosis and kyphosis, are only important if they are quite advanced. Leg length inequality also seems to be important only if the discrepancy is quite large. This obviously does not mean that these conditions should not be treated as indicated.

Height, weight, and body build are believed to be of minor importance. Back

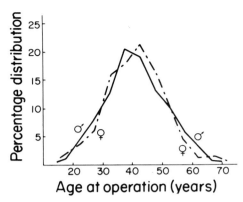

FIG. 4. Percentage distribution of operations for herniated lumbar discs by age and sex. (Adapted from Spangfort (1972), with permission.)

pain is more common in the very tall and in the very obese. However, within large ranges, height and weight are probably unimportant. Physical strength is a risk factor only if work demands are such that they approach the maximum strength of the worker. And even so the predictive value in terms of injury risk remains uncertain. Physical fitness, as such, seems to be important primarily as a factor hastening recovery after a back pain episode, while spine mobility is decreased when back pain exists, but doesn't seem to be a predictor of future risk. Fitness is associated with other lifestyle factors that may influence the risk of back pain as well. This is also true for smoking. Smokers have an increased risk of back pain in many studies. This may be due to repetitive strain, but smoking also decreases the oxygen tension in spinal tissues, such as the disc, and increases the risk of disc degeneration.

Heredity plays a minor role in back disorders. Thus, common low back and neck syndromes seem to be caused mainly by environmental factors, although a familial predisposition to adolescent disc herniations has been reported.

OTHER RISK FACTORS IN BACK PAIN

A history of back symptoms is a strong indicator of future risk. This is particularly the case if the previous symptoms were severe, occurred frequently, or required surgical treatment. This is understandable considering that recurrences are part of the natural history of back problems.

Degenerative changes in the spine are common and should be considered part of the aging process, not indicators of disease entities as such. Traumatic injuries and heavy physical loading lead to earlier and more severe degenerative changes, as do spinal deformities.

Disability from back pain is influenced by a variety of factors, including culture, socioeconomic conditions, compensation, emotional distress, job satisfaction, work environment, and treatment. Unfortunately, there is evidence that disability caused by back pain is increasing, in spite of significant efforts in terms of prevention.

THE NATURAL HISTORY OF LOW BACK PAIN

The natural history of low back pain is excellent. Patients should be expected to recover from an acute episode in 3 to 4 wk and often recover in a few days to 1 wk (Fig. 5). Recovery from sciatica is somewhat slower on average, mainly because some patients with sciatica have a more severe underlying problem (such as a disc hernia or spinal stenosis). About

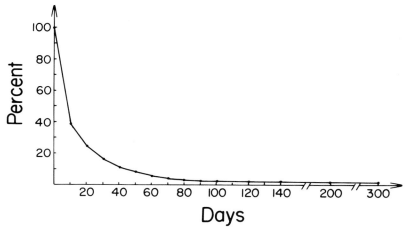

FIG. 5. Proportion of patients still sick-listed as a function of time. Note the rapid return to work and the small percentage still absent after 60 days. (Adapted from Andersson et al. (1983), with permission.)

50% of patients with disc hernia–induced sciatica will recover spontaneously in 4 to 6 wk. A small percentage of all patients with back pain develop chronic symptoms. Factors contributing to chronic back pain include severe underlying disorder, psychosocial dysfunction, and work-related factors. Old age and poor physical condition are other factors increasing the risk of chronicity. Iatrogenic factors such as a recommendation for long-term bed rest and passive treatment modalities contribute to the prolongation of recovery, as discussed in later chapters. Although recovery is typically fast, back pain tends to recur from time to time. Over 50% of patients who have an acute episode of low back pain will have another episode within a year.

Surgery is seldom necessary. The lifetime incidence of surgery for back pain and sciatica ranges from 1% to 3%. Surgery hastens the recovery from disc hernia–induced sciatica but seems to have little influence on risk of recurrence.

The natural history of neck pain is similarly excellent, with expected spontaneous recovery in days to weeks. Surgery for cervical disc herniations is much less frequent than for lumbar herniations, again occurs more often among patients who are 40 to 50 years old, and is more frequent among heavy industrial workers.

THE COST OF BACK PAIN

Because of its prevalence and demand on health care, back pain is one of the most expensive disease entities. Although we cannot precisely determine the total cost, a reasonable estimate for direct cost in 1990 in the United States alone is $23.5 billion. Indirect costs (i.e., the value of output lost because of cessation or reduction in productivity) are probably at least of the same magnitude. They are so difficult to predict, however, that the overall cost of spinal disorders to U.S. society is variably estimated at $25 billion to $100 billion. The figure for all nations would obviously be several times higher.

SUGGESTED READING

1. Andersson GBJ, Svensson H-O, Oden A. The intensity of work recovery in low back pain. *Spine* 1983;8:880–884.
2. Biering-Sorensen F. Low back trouble in a general population of 30-, 40-, 50- and 60-year old men and women. *Dan Med Bull* 1982;29 (6):289–299.
3. Deyo RA, Tsui-Wu Y-J. Descriptive epidemiology of low-back pain and its related medical care in the United States. *Spine* 1987; 12:264–268.
4. Frymoyer JW. *The adult spine.* New York: Raven Press; 1991. A major treatise on adult spinal conditions. Epidemiologic aspects are covered in Chapters 7, 8, 9, and 70.
5. Klein BP, Jensen RC, Sanderson LM. Assessment of workers' compensation claims for back strains/sprains. *J Occup Med* 1984;26:443–448.
6. Pope MH, Andersson GBJ, Frymoyer JW, Chaffin DB. *Occupational low back pain: assessment, treatment and prevention.* St. Louis: Mosby Year Book; 1991. A book that covers all aspects of the back problem in industry. Epidemiology is covered in Chapters 5, 6, 7, and 13.
7. Praemer A, Furner S, Rice DP. *Musculoskeletal conditions in the United States.* Park Ridge: American Academy of Orthopaedic Surgeons; 1992. A summary of the prevalence and incidence of musculoskeletal conditions in the United States.
8. Spangfort EV. The lumbar disc herniation. *Acta Orthop Scand Suppl* 1972;142:1–95.

2

Classification and Pathophysiology of Spinal Pain Syndromes

Kjell Olmarker and *Mitsuo Hasue

*Department of Orthopaedics, Sahlgren University Hospital,
S-413 45 Gothenburg, Sweden; and *Department of Orthopedic Surgery,
Japanese Red Cross Medical Center, Tokyo, Japan*

Key Points

- Low back pain is a very common condition, but in most patients the origin of pain is not known.

- Spinal pain may be classified based on the onset/duration or the location/radiation.

- Pain in the lumbar spine is called *low back pain* or *lumbago*. Pain radiating into the leg according to the distribution of one or several nerve roots is called *sciatica*. A common cause of sciatica is disc herniation.

- Neurogenic claudication is a special condition with pain or numbness in the legs at exercise, such as walking. The underlying pathologic condition for such symptoms is usually spinal stenosis.

Spinal pain syndromes are one of the largest socioeconomic problems of modern society. For instance, in Sweden as much as $3 billion (U.S.) were spent in 1990 for diagnosis, treatment, and rehabilitation of spinal pain syndromes. The spinal pain syndromes also constitute one of the most intriguing medical conditions, as little is known about the exact pathophysiologic mechanisms involved. Many mechanisms have been suggested, but scientific confirmation is still, to a large extent, nonexistent. Current treatment modalities are thus based on experience rather than on a scientific basis. To understand why knowledge about the etiology and pathophysiology of spinal pain syndromes is so limited, one must consider that spinal pain is a symptom rather than a specific disease. It would thus be just as pointless to look for one specific mechanism for spinal pain as it would be to look for one specific mechanism for another unspecific reaction, for instance, headache or fever. Thus, spinal pain is a general symptom that may be based on a variety of different etiologic and pathophysiologic mechanisms. However, spinal pain may be experienced in terms of onset, duration, and localization. It may, therefore, be possible to classify spinal pain in such a way to obtain some guidelines regarding which pathophysiologic mechanisms may be present for a given individual.

THE CLASSIFICATION OF SPINAL PAIN

One way to classify spinal pain syndromes is by onset and duration (Table 1). If pain has an immediate onset and the duration is less than 3 mo, it may be called *acute*. However, if the onset is somewhat more gradual, with a duration of less than 3 mo, it is referred to as *subacute*. If the duration is more than 3 mo, regardless of onset, it is called *chronic*. If there is an

TABLE 1. *Classification of spinal pain—onset/duration*

Acute pain	Immediate onset, with a duration of 0 to 3 mo
Subacute pain	Slow onset, with a duration of 0 to 3 mo
Chronic pain	More than 3 mo in duration
Recurring pain	Symptoms recurring after an interval of no symptoms

Modified from Nachemson and Andersson (1982), with permission.

TABLE 2. *Classification of spinal pain—location/radiation*

Local pain	Pain is located at the lower lumbar or lumbosacral area and is usually called low back pain.
Referred pain	Pain is located at the area that shares a common embryologic origin with the region involved (myotomes and sclerotomes considered). A synonym for this pain is sclerotomal pain.
Radicular pain	Pain is located along the dermatomal distribution of a spinal nerve root. It may be accompanied by sensory and motor deficits. A synonym is dermatomal pain.

interval of no symptoms but pain reappears, it is called *recurrent* pain.

Another way to classify pain is by location and distribution (radiation) (Table 2). Pain originating from the lumbar spine may be classified into three categories—local, referred, and radicular pain. *Local pain,* also called low back pain and/or lumbago, is located at the lower lumbar or lumbosacral area. *Referred pain* is experienced at the area that shares a common embryologic origin with the region involved. It is usually located to the inguinal or buttock region and/or the anterior, lateral, or posterior thigh. In some cases, however, it might be distributed even below the knee. *Radicular pain* is distributed along the dermatomal distribution of a spinal nerve root and is due to a direct affection of the nerve tissue (Fig. 1). It is most commonly experienced along the course of the sciatic nerve depending on the spinal level of the involved nerve root.

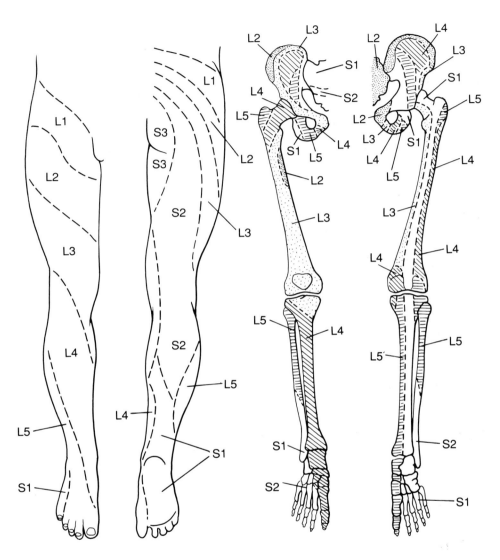

FIG. 1. To the *left* is the dermatomal distribution of the innervation by each nerve root level demonstrated. To the *right* is the corresponding sclerotomal innervation. (Modified from Inman and Saunders (1944), with permission.)

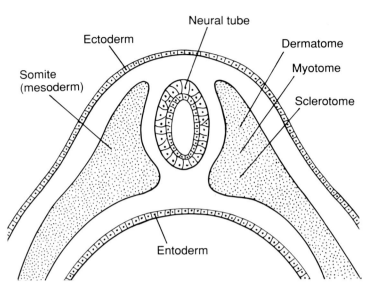

FIG. 2. The middle layer (mesoderm) in this 21-day-old fetus has formed a somite. This somite represents one future nerve root level and will later be transformed into a dermatome, a myotome, and a sclerotome.

Neurogenic intermittent claudication due to lumbar spine disorders is a unique symptom that should be distinguished from the pain types presented in Tables 1 and 2 and will be discussed later.

PATHOANATOMIC CONSIDERATIONS

In early embryonic stages, the body is formed by three layers of undifferentiated tissue called *ectoderm, mesoderm,* and *entoderm* (Fig. 2). The mesoderm forms about 30 to 36 somites that will later be differentiated into dermatomes, myotomes, and sclerotomes (Fig. 2). Each somite represents one nerve root level. The dermatome will form the inner layer of the skin, and its innervation is equivalent to

the dermatomal innervation of the skin (Fig. 1). The myotome will form the muscles, and each muscle will have an innervation that can be referred to a specific nerve root level. This innervation pattern is called *myotomal innervation* (Table 3). The myotome of a specific nerve root may thus be tested by testing either the muscular strength or the reflexes (Table 3). A deficit in both the myotome and the dermatome for one nerve root supports the assumption that this nerve root may be involved. The sclerotomes will form connective structures, such as bone and cartilage. As with the muscles, the different parts of the skeleton have innervations that may be related to specific nerve roots; this is called *sclerotomal innervation* (Fig. 1). The sclerotomal distribution is quite dif-

TABLE 3. *Myotomes related to spinal pain syndromes*

Root	Muscle	Function	Reflex
L4	M quadriceps femoris	Knee extension	Patellar
L5	M tib. ant./M ext. hall. long.	Dorsiflexion of foot/great toe	None valid
S1	M gastrocnemius	Plantar flexion of foot	Achilles

ferent from the dermatomal distribution. Referred pain due to involvement of the 4th lumbar through 1st sacral nerve root levels usually results in a dull pain at the region of the hip and the femur rather than radiating pain into the legs. One of the reasons might be related to the fact that the sclerotomal innervation of axons originating from those nerve roots is more compactly located in the above-knee area.

Local (Low Back) Pain

There is a general opinion that low back pain is due to local affections in the supporting structures of the lumbar spine such as muscles, tendons, ligaments, facet joints, and intervertebral discs. There is probably no reason to believe that any structure in the spinal canal would be involved. Theoretically, any structure with pain receptors in the lumbar spine may be involved in the production of low back pain.

Referred Pain

This type of pain is, as described previously, related to the embryologic origin of the structures such as facet joints, ligaments, and intervertebral discs in the lumbar spine and in the lower extremities. The site of pain production is the peripheral *somatic* tissue. The pain is transmitted by the nerve and localized to a specific nerve root level. In this regard,

the myotomes and sclerotomes are of importance. This type of referred pain is called *somatosomatic* and is important in bone and joint diseases. Another form of referred pain is *viscerosomatic,* where pain in a visceral organ such as the heart may present as somatic pain. For instance, the pain from the heart is typically located into the left arm.

Radicular Pain

Pain is related to the spinal nerve root per se. The nerve root is compressed or irritated in the lumbar spine, and pain may be directly related to a specific nerve root level. It is not uncommon that sensory and/or motor deficit is present and corresponds to the involved nerve root. This pain should be distinguished from referred pain.

Sciatica

Sciatica has been known to exist for many hundred years. The term *sciatica* literally means "related to the hip." However, the first time the word *sciatica* is found in the literature is not in a scientific paper but in a play "Timons of Athens" by William Shakespeare, where the character Timon cries out, "Thou could sciatica, cripples our senators as lamely as their manners." The first pathoanatomic definition of sciatica was made by

Domenico Cortugno, who in 1576 stated that sciatica was a local affection of the sciatic nerve in the thigh. However, it was yet another 325 yr, at the turn of the 20th century, until independent authors reported that leg pain could be the result of injury to the spinal nerve roots in the lumbar spine. In 1929, Dandy reported the existence of chondromas, or cartilage tumors, arising from the intervertebral discs and compressing the nerve roots, with subsequent sciatic pain. The same year, Schmorl, a German radiologist, demonstrated the presence of disc herniations. These disc herniations were present in all directions from the disc. However, only the herniations penetrating into adjacent vertebrae, today known as *nodules of Schmorl,* were considered to be of clinical importance. It was some 5 yr until Mixter and Barr for the first time presented the relationship between sciatica and the presence of an intraspinal herniation of the soft, central substance of the disc called the *nucleus pulposus.* Since then, compression of a spinal nerve root by herniated disc material has been considered to be the direct cause of sciatica.

Neurogenic Intermittent Claudication

Intermittent claudication has generally been attributed to an occlusive vascular disease of the legs. In the mid-1950s, however, Verbiest linked this clinical picture also to a narrowing of the spinal canal, or *spinal stenosis,* with subsequent compression of the spinal nerve roots. Typically, the patient can walk a certain distance until such leg symptoms as pain, numbness, or dullness appear and force the patient to stop walking. After a while, usually after taking a semi-flexed or sitting position, the patient can once again start to walk. This specific condition was named *neurogenic intermittent claudication.*

PATHOPHYSIOLOGIC MECHANISMS

Pain receptors have been found in a large number of tissues related to the spine. Thus, one may assume that practically all structures in the spine may be involved in the production of pain in some way. However, some structures seem to be more likely to produce pain than are others.

Regarding superficial support structures such as skin, fascia, muscle, and ligaments, it is not unreasonable to assume that these structures may produce local pain if injured or overused. This is a common phenomenon in other parts of the body, for instance in the upper and lower extremities, and we have reason to believe that it should not be any different in the spine. Likewise, the periosteum and joint capsules in the extremities are known to produce pain if exposed to excessive stress or injury. The same thing should be applicable in the spine, with its periosteum and facet joint capsules. Studies have been performed where unanesthetized spinal structures have been stimulated mechanically either during progressive local anesthesia or after surgery by pulling ligatures attached to intraspinal structures. Structures such as annulus fibrosus, vertebral endplate, ante-

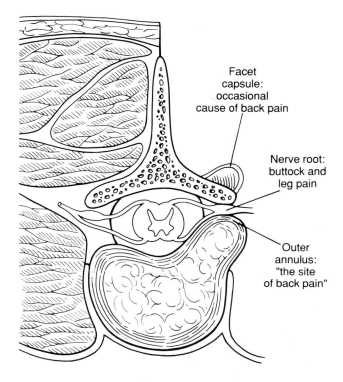

FIG. 3. Different structures of the spine will produce pain when stimulated intraoperatively. (Modified from Kuslich et al. (1991), with permission.)

rior dura, posterior longitudinal ligament, and facet capsules induce various degrees of pain localized in the lumbar spine (Fig. 3). Mechanical stimulation of nonirritated nerve roots did not induce any pain. However, stimulation of nerve roots exposed to herniated disc material, which were often irritated, produced an intense pain response that usually radiated out into the leg and foot on the corresponding side.

There is probably another situation when the intraspinal nervous structures are involved (Fig. 4). Usually pain is the result of a stimulation of some kind of receptor that will transmit the pain through specific fibers to the spinal cord and then further to the brain, where it might be perceived as pain. However, a direct stimulation or irritation of the nerve somewhere between its receptor and the brain may result in a similar pain perception. The pain in this case cannot be localized to the irritation site but rather is referred to the receptor site. This is probably the mechanism for nerve root compression in the lumbar spine with sciatica, where a nerve root containing axons from the leg is compressed, but the pain is not localized to the lumbar spine but

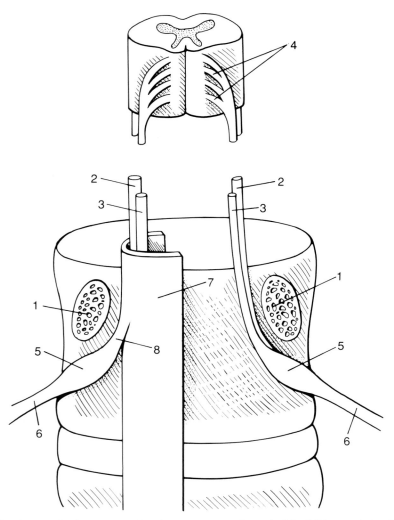

FIG. 4. The intraspinal nervous structures as seen from behind. The vertebral arches are removed by cutting the pedicles (*1*). A ventral (*2*) and a dorsal (*3*) nerve root leave the spinal cord as small rootlets (*4*). Before leaving the spinal canal, the dorsal root forms a swelling called the *dorsal root ganglion* (*5*), which contains the sensory cell bodies, before forming the spinal nerve (*6*) together with the ventral nerve root. The nerve roots are covered by a central dural sac (*7*) or with extensions of this sac called *nerve root sleeves* (*8*). (From Olmarker (1990), with permission.)

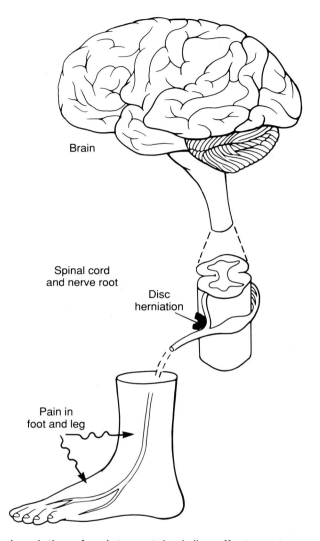

FIG. 5. When a herniation of an intervertebral disc affects a nerve root in the lumbar spine, the brain may interpret the pain as coming from the end of the axons involved (i.e., from the foot and leg).

to the receptor site of the compressed axons in the leg (Fig. 5).

Exactly what happens when a nerve, or nerve root, is exposed to a herniated disc or a narrowing of the spinal canal is not known. Numerous experimental studies on the effects of compression on peripheral nerves (i.e., nerves outside the spinal canal—for instance, in the extremities) have shown that there is both a

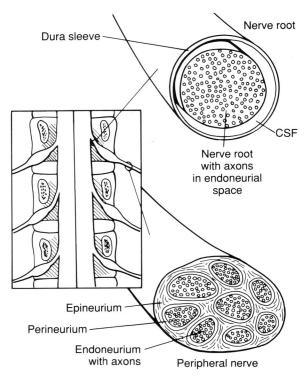

FIG. 6. In the spinal canal the nerve roots are covered by the cerebrospinal fluid (CSF) and a dural sleeve. However, after leaving the spinal canal, the axons are split to smaller fascicles and covered by the perineurium and the epineurium. These two structures will protect the axons from mechanical deformation and are more pronounced where the nerve is at risk, as, for instance, when a nerve is running close to a joint.

mechanical component, with deformation of the nerve tissue, and a reduction of the blood flow within the nerve and therefore the nutrition to the nerve. These two effects are very difficult to separate, but blood flow reduction is considered to appear at a pressure in the region of 30 to 50 mm Hg. Mechanical deformation, however, does not develop until exposure to pressure exceeds 200 mm Hg. These data cannot be directly transferred to the spinal nerve roots since they have a less well-developed protective anatomic arrangement of connective tissue (Fig. 6). It seems that these structures are so well protected by the surrounding vertebrae that they have not developed the protective connective tissue layers necessary for peripheral nerves, which are much less protected in the extremities. Recent studies have established new critical pressure levels for inducing nerve injury in the spinal nerve roots. These studies indicate that the nerve roots are far more susceptible to nerve injury. Blood flow and nutritional transport begins to be impaired at

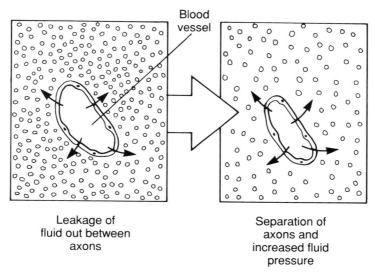

Leakage of
fluid out between
axons

Separation of
axons and
increased fluid
pressure

FIG. 7. If the permeability of an intraneural capillary is increased, there may be a leakage of fluid and macromolecules to the axons. This results in a separation of the axons and an increased fluid pressure. This situation is called *intraneural edema* and may significantly affect the normal function of the nerve.

pressures of 5 to 10 mm Hg. Functional impairment may be seen at 75 to 100 mm Hg compression for 2 hr, but there are indications that significant impairment may be seen also at 5 to 10 mm Hg if prolonged for days or weeks. As a secondary effect to the nutritional deficit induced by compression, intraneural edema may develop in the nerve root. This means that fluid leaks out from the intraneural blood vessels into the axons in the endoneurial space (Fig. 7). This may increase the fluid pressure around the axons and in this way reduce the normal flow of nutrients and metabolic waste products between the axons and the blood vessels.

The peripheral nerves in the extremities have a continuous supply of regional arteries and veins. This is not the case for nerve roots, which lack these connecting vessels (Fig. 8). This means that, if a nerve root is compressed at two different locations, there will be a nutritional deficit in all parts of the nerve root located between the two compression sites. This has recently been confirmed experimentally, and it has also been shown clinically that patients with double-level compression usually have more aggravated symptoms than do patients with compression at only one level.

It is difficult to assess pain in the various experimental models. Usually one has to rely on such indirect information as registration of nerve impulses from axons of a certain size that are known to transmit impulses that are interpreted as pain by the brain. However, recently established techniques allow for determination of concentration and synthesis rates of certain neuropeptides that are

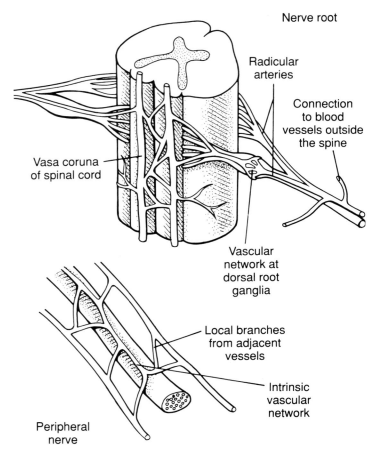

FIG. 8. The vascular supply to the nerve root comes from the spinal cord and peripherally from blood vessels outside the spine. Radicular arteries are formed and supply the nerve root from both directions. The nerve root has no connections to surrounding vessels. In the peripheral nerve, however, the vascular system of the nerve has numerous connections to surrounding vessels along its course.

related to the axonal transmission of pain. Two neuropeptides that are supposed to be related to such pain transmission are Substance P and vasointestinal peptide (VIP). With such techniques it has recently been established that vibration and mild compression and/or irritation of nerve roots may induce an increase in both concentration and synthesis rates.

Such changes have particularly been noted in the dorsal root ganglion, which contains the sensory cell bodies where these peptides are synthesized.

In some patients with clinically apparent sciatica associated with pain and neurologic dysfunction related to one specific spinal nerve root segment, it has been observed that there is no compression of

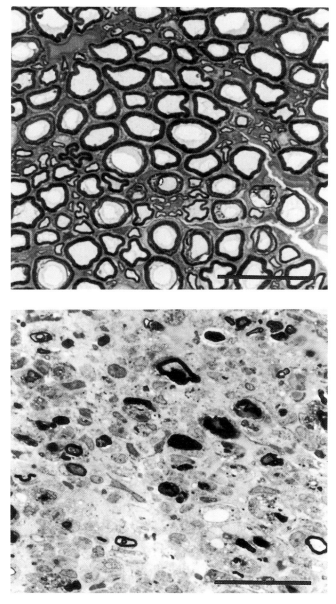

FIG. 9. At the *top* is a normal nerve root from a pig. The axons are seen as white irregular dots and are surrounded by the black myelin sheath. At the *bottom* is a pig nerve root that has been exposed to normal nucleus pulposus from the same animal. Compared to the picture on the *top,* one cannot distinguish any axons or myelin. There is a severe nerve injury present with ongoing degeneration of the axons. *Bars* in both pictures are 100 μm.

the nerve root, neither by radiologic examination or at surgery. It has therefore been assumed that other factors than compression might be present. One possible mechanism suggested is that some of the various components in the nucleus pulposus of the intervertebral disc might affect the nerve root in some way. This could be either by a direct irritative or toxic effect or by an indirect effect of the vascularization of the nerve root. Since the nucleus pulposus is nonvascularized itself and thus hidden from the immunologic defense system of the body, it has also been suggested that leakage of nucleus pulposus might induce an immunologic reaction directed against the nucleus pulposus, which is considered to be foreign material once presented to the immune system. Such a reaction is called *autoimmune* as it implies an immunologic reaction to tissues from the same body. However, only recently have theories related to an effect of the nucleus pulposus been demonstrated experimentally. Local application of autologous nucleus pulposus (i.e., from the same animal) on the nerve roots, without any compression, has been shown to induce significant reduction in nerve conduction velocity and significant histologic changes in the nerve fibers themselves (Fig. 9). Autologous nucleus pulposus also seems to possess certain inflammatogenic properties, meaning that, when applied somewhere in the same body, an inflammatory reaction is induced. At present, however, it is not evident whether such a reaction is a true autoimmune response, whether this is merely due to mechanical irritation, or whether there are inflammatory mediators in the disc. Both human phospholipase A2 and interleukin-6, which are two potent inflammatogenic substances, have now been identified in the associated herniated nucleus pulposus. However, several studies demonstrate progress in this new field of research. It is not unlikely that this research may eventually provide results that could be used for newly developed diagnostic and therapeutic modalities.

CONCLUDING REMARKS

Spinal pain is a symptom that may have different causes. It is one of the most costly and intriguing medical conditions today. For the individual patient, there is often a very good prognosis. A majority of all patients are fully recovered within weeks after onset. This chapter has discussed a classification system and has provided a limited review of the current knowledge of the basic mechanisms behind various conditions associated with spinal pain. However, the research in this field is very active and in the near future there may be new possibilities to facilitate the diagnosis and treatment of various spinal pain syndromes.

SUGGESTED READING

1. Bobechko WP, Hirsch C. Auto-immune response to nucleus pulposus in the rabbit. *J Bone Joint Surg [Br]*1965;47B:574–580.
2. Chatani K, Kawakami M, Weinstein JN, Meller ST, Gebhart GF. Characterization of thermal hyperalgesia, C-fos expression and alterations in neuropeptides following mechanical irritation of the dorsal root ganglion. *Spine* 1995;20(3).
3. De Silva M, Hazleman BL, Ward M, Park JR, Dickson I. Auto-immunity and the prolapsed intervertebral disc syndrome. *Reumatologie* 1981;1:35–38.

4. Feinstein B, Langton JNK, Jameson RM, Schiller F. Experiments on pain referred from deep somatic tissues. *J Bone Joint Surg [Am]* 1954;36A:981–997.

5. Gertzbein SD, Tile M, Gross A, Falk R. Autoimmunity in degenerative disc disease of the lumbar spine. *Orthop Clin North Am* 1975;6:67–73.

6. Gertzbein SD. Degenerative disk disease of the lumbar spine: immunological implications. *Clin Orthop* 1977;129:69–71.

7. Inman VT, Saunders JBC. Referred pain from skeletal structures. *J Nerve Ment Dis* 1944; 99:660–667.

8. Kawakami M, Weinstein JN, Chatani K, Spratt KF, Meller ST, Gebhart GF. Experimental lumbar radiculopathy: behavioral and histological changes in a model of radicular pain after spinal nerve root irritation with chronic gut ligatures in the rat. Part II. *Spine* 1994;19(16):1795–1802.

9. Kawakami M, Weinstein JN, Spratt KF, Chatani K, Gebhart GF, Traub RJ, Meller ST. Experimental lumbar radiculopathy: immunohistochemical and quantitative demonstrations of pain induced by lumbar nerve root irritation of the rat. Part I. AcroMed Award Paper. *Spine* 1994;19(16):1780–1794.

10. Kelly M. Is pain due to pressure of nerves? *Neurology* 1956;6:32–36.

11. Kuslich SD, Ulstrom CL, Michael CJ. The tissue origin of low back pain and sciatica. *Orthop Clin North Am* 1991;22:181–187.

12. LaRocca H. New horizons in research on disc disease. *Orthop Clin North Am* 1971;2:521.

13. Marshall LL, Trethewie ER. Chemical irritation of nerve-root in disc prolapse. *Lancet* 1973;2:320.

14. Marshall LL, Trethewie ER, Curtain CC. Chemical radiculitis. *Clin Orthop* 1977;129: 61–67.

15. McCarron RF, Wimpee MW, Hudkins P, Laros GS. The inflammatory effect of nucleus pulposus: a possible element in the pathogenesis of low-back pain. *Spine* 1987;12:760–764.

16. Mixter WJ, Barr JS. Rupture of the intervertebral disc with involvement of the spinal canal. *N Engl J Med* 1934;211:210–215.

17. Nachemson AL. The lumbar spine, an orthopaedic challenge. *Spine* 1976;1:59–71.

18. Nachemson AL, Andersson GBJ Classification of low-back pain. *Scand J Work Environ Health* 1982;134–136.

19. Olmarker K. *Spinal nerve root compression* [Thesis]. Gothenburg, Sweden: Gothenburg University, 1990.

20. Olmarker K. Spinal nerve root compression: nutrition and function of the porcine cauda equina compressed in vivo. *Acta Orthop Scand Suppl* 1991;242.

21. Olmarker K, Rydevik B. Single versus double level compression: an experimental study on the porcine cauda equina with analyses of nerve impulse conduction properties. *Clin Orthop* 1992;279:35–39.

22. Olmarker K, Rydevik B, Nordborg C. Autologous nucleus pulposus induces neurophysiologic and histologic changes in porcine cauda equina nerve roots. *Spine* 1993; 18:1425–1432.

23. Porter RW, Ward D. Cauda equina dysfunction. The significance of two-level pathology. *Spine* 1992;17:9–15.

24. Rydevik BL, Pedowitz RA, Hargens AR, Swenson MR, Myers RR, Garfin SR. Effects of acute graded compression on spinal nerve root function and structure: an experimental study on the pig cauda equina. *Spine* 1991; 16:487–493.

25. Saal JS, Franson RC, Dobrow R, Saal JA, White AH, Goldthwaite N. High levels of inflammatory phospholipase A2 activity in lumbar disc herniations. *Spine* 1990;15: 674–678.

26. Schmorl G. Über knorpelknoten an der hinterfläche der Wirbelbandscheiben. *Fortschr Geb Rontgenstr* 1926.

27. Smyth MJ, Wright V. Sciatica and the intervertebral disc: an experimental study. *J Bone Joint Surg [Am]* 1958;40A:1401–1418.

28. Verbiest H. A radicular syndrome from developmental narrowing of the lumbar spine vertebral canal. *J Bone Joint Surg [Br]* 1954; 36B:230–237.

29. Weinstein J. Mechanism of spinal pain: the dorsal root ganglion and its role as a mediator of low back pain. *Spine* 1986;11:999–1001.

30. Weinstein JN, Pope M, Schmidt R, et al. The effects of low frequency vibration on dorsal root ganglion Substance P. *Neuro-orthopaedics* 1987;4:24–30.

31. Weinstein JN, Pope M, Schmidt R, Seroussi R. Neuropharmacologic effects of vibration on the dorsal root ganglion—an animal model. *Spine* 1988;13(5):521–525.

3
Pathology of Spinal Disorders

Richard W. Porter

Department of Orthopaedic Surgery, Aberdeen University,
AB9 2ZD Aberdeen, United Kingdom

Key Points

- Back pain is a symptom, not a diagnosis.

- Mechanical low back pain is the most common type of back pain.

- Differential diagnosis includes specific causes such as spondylolisthesis, tumor, and inflammatory conditions, as well as nonspinal causes such as gynecologic, renal, and intestinal disorders.

- Lumbar disc herniation and spinal stenosis exhibit different clinical symptoms.

- There are three important aspects of each vertebral fracture: (a) Is the spine stable or unstable? (b) Are there neurologic symptoms and signs? (c) Is the back pain likely to be temporary or chronic?

To understand the natural history, we need a diagnosis. Back pain is a symptom, not a diagnosis, and the pathologic condition may not even be in the spine. The differential diagnosis of back pain includes many nonspinal causes. These are gynecologic, renal, pancreatic, gallbladder disease, subphrenic abscess, aortic aneurysm, posterior duodenal ulcer, and retroperitoneal fibrosis. The periodicity of pain from these sites is related to the system of origin.

Abnormalities in the vertebral body include metastases, primary bone tumors, cordoma, multiple myelomatosis, leukemia, acute osteomyelitis, tuberculosis, brucellosis, and discitis. The pain is usually constant, often with systematic disturbance.

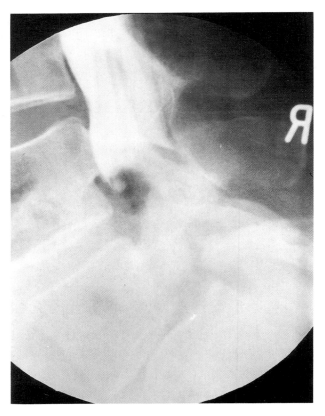

FIG. 1. Lateral myelogram showing an intradural tumor, a rare paraganglionoma. The diagnosis was delayed because the symptoms were thought to be due to the isthmic spondylolisthesis at L-5.

Spinal tumor may be intradural or extradural with bizarre symptoms and signs, causing delay in making the diagnosis (Fig. 1). Inflammatory causes are ankylosing spondylitis (Figs. 2 and 3), sacral ileitis, psoriasis, and Reiter's disease. Pain is usually worse after rest, with morning stiffness. Pain often alternates between one side of the back and the other.

Mechanical back pain is the commonest cause of back pain and the subject of this book. By definition, it is a pain in the back precipitated by and aggravated by mechanical factors. There are two types: First, low back pain, with or without referred pain but not nerve root pain. Pain that is referred from the spine is experienced in the buttock or the thigh and occasionally below the knee. There is no root abnormality, but the nociceptive source in the spine is interpreted centrally as being pain referred to a distance. The pain in the back is usually worse than the pain referred to the distant site. Second, in nerve root pathologic conditions the symptoms extend in a root distribution,

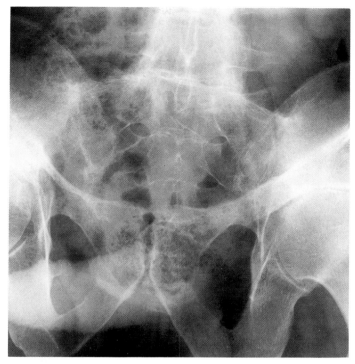

FIG. 2. Anteroposterior (AP) radiograph of the pelvis of a 42-yr-old man with an 18-yr history of ankylosing spondylitis, showing sacroiliac joint fusion and degenerative changes of the hips.

often in the buttock, thigh, or calf to the ankle and sometimes with pins and needles in the foot. The distribution of L3 root pain, however, may be confused with referred pain. Root pain in the leg is worse than the pain in the back.

LOW BACK PAIN OF MECHANICAL ORIGIN WITH OR WITHOUT REFERRED PAIN

The pathologic process in acute low back pain is difficult to define. Ligaments or muscles can be strained, or the facet joint disturbed. However, the most common cause is an acute disc protrusion (Fig. 4), which causes bulging of the posterior annulus and will often present initially as acute low back pain, sometimes referred into the buttock or thigh. The peripheral annulus has pain-sensitive nerves and when stretched can be responsible for acute low back pain. There are few signs, however, that will distinguish this nociceptive source from other types of mechanical back pain. Sometimes only in retrospect when a patient has nerve root pain from a disc sequestration will the earlier onset of back pain be attributed to a bulging annulus.

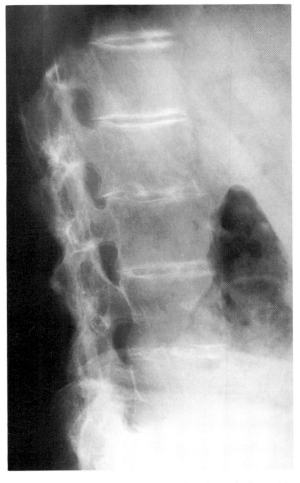

FIG. 3. Lateral radiograph of the same patient's ankylosed lumbar spine.

In chronic low back pain, the pathologic condition is even more difficult to determine. When low back pain becomes chronic, it is difficult to determine its cause. Chronic motion segment failure can be associated with chronic low back pain. The motion segment is a three-joint system composed of the intervertebral disc and the two apophyseal joints. Degeneration of one component affects the other two, with disc degeneration usu-ally preceding apophyseal joint arthritis. There are two possible mechanisms of the motion segment becoming painful. The first is pain associated with excessive or erratic motion, with the nociceptive source being the apophyseal joint, the capsule, the ligaments, or the annulus (Fig. 5). Muscle or ligamentous fatigue may be a source of pain when the soft tissues fail to restrain abnormal motion. A second possible source of pain

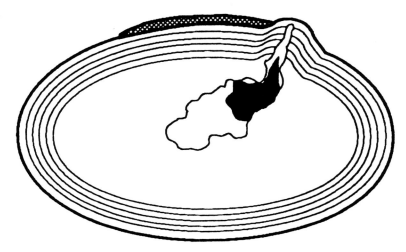

FIG. 4. Diagram to show a disc protrusion, with a fragment of disc causing the annulus to bulge.

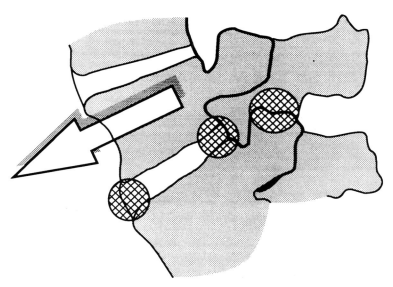

FIG. 5. Nociceptive source in structures restraining erratic or excessive motion (muscles, ligaments, joint capsule, outer annulus).

in the failed motion segment can be the vertebral endplate, which may be pain sensitive to loading (Fig. 6). Many patients with motion segment failure experience their first symptoms in pregnancy, possibly when there is an already degenerated disc that is aggravated by abnormal mechanics and the circulating hormone, relaxin.

Isthmic spondylolisthesis results from defects in the pars interarticularis and can be responsible for episodic or chronic low back pain. Degenerative spondylolisthesis, however, usually occurs at the L4-5 level when the 4th lumbar vertebra displaces forward with an intact neural arch. It is usually responsible for chronic low back pain, often associated with neurologic compromise from stenosis of the central canal or root canal.

It is important to understand the natural history of low back pain. When it is associated with a bulging annulus, the symptoms usually develop suddenly and the pain can be quite severe, but it generally settles over a few days or weeks, often completely. There may be only one or two episodes in a lifetime or frequent episodes of acute back pain, steadily increasing in severity. Ultimately, the disc may herniate, leaving a sequestrated fragment adjacent to the nerve root and producing severe root pain. Thus, the natural history can be quite variable, and it is often only when the patient has root pathology that the diagnosis is confirmed.

The natural history of motion segment failure is also variable, but most patients tend to experience chronic back pain, varying in degree for a number of years. The pain frequently begins in middle life, but in old age it is less of a problem. This may be because degenerative change is sometimes beneficial, stabilizing a segment. In addition, the demands on the spine decrease with age. There may be an altered pain mechanism in the elderly. The silent myocardial infarct or perforated peptic ulcer and the elderly man with a grossly distended bladder from prostatic hypertrophy suggest that the experience of pain can be modified in the elderly. Age can be kindly to the spine.

The prognosis in isthmic spondylolisthesis is quite variable. The first episode of pain can be acute and then settle down, the pain can be episodic, or it can create a chronic disability, but generally it becomes less troublesome in old age.

Pain associated with degenerative spondylolisthesis, however, once established tends to persist and be a chronic problem. Symptoms first occur in patients over 45 yr of age, generally in women at the L4-5 level.

THE PROLAPSED INTERVERTEBRAL DISC

The first symptoms of disc protrusion are preceded by months or years of symptomless disease. When symptoms occur, however, they depend on a disc fragment compressing a nerve root in a small canal, and there are also probably biochemical factors (Fig. 7).

The texture of the intervertebral disc changes with age, gradually losing water content from 90% in early adult life to 70% in the elderly. The gross morphology of the disc, however, can remain intact throughout life. A considerable proportion of discs develop fissures that are not necessarily symptomatic. Prolapse of

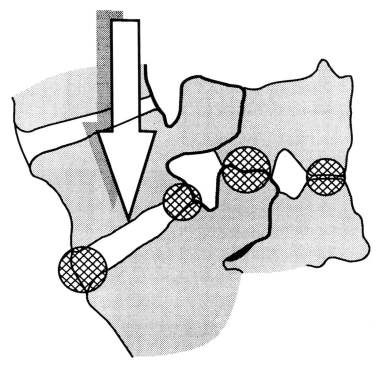

FIG. 6. Nociceptive source in structures bearing load (annulus, apophyseal joints, spinous process).

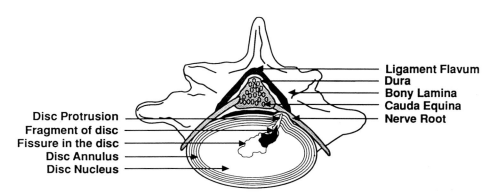

Ligament Flavum
Dura
Bony Lamina
Cauda Equina
Nerve Root

Disc Protrusion
Fragment of disc
Fissure in the disc
Disc Annulus
Disc Nucleus

FIG. 7. Diagram showing how a loose fragment of the nucleus pulposus can cause an annular bulge compressing a nerve root against the bony lamina.

an intervertebral disc occurs when there is not only a fissure but also a fragment within the disc. Laboratory studies have shown that creating an experimental fissure in a cadaveric disc and loading the segment will not produce a protrusion. But if a loose fragment from another disc is introduced into the fissure, then, with very low physiologic loads, the fragment can be squeezed backward toward the posterior annulus like a "pea in a pod." The annulus will bulge and quickly herniate through an extension of the fissure, tearing through the posterior annulus. A disc protrusion occurs when the annulus is bulging but intact. A disc sequestration occurs when a loose fragment herniates through a complete tear in the annulus to lie free within the vertebral canal. Twenty percent of asymptomatic subjects will have a disc protrusion or sequestration by 60 years of age.

Whether a patient experiences root symptoms in association with a disc protrusion depends on the available space within the vertebral canal. Fifty percent of patients who are admitted with root symptoms and signs from a disc protrusion have vertebral canal measurements in the bottom tenth percentile of canal size. Subjects with wider canals may have a protrusion, but they avoid root problems. The nerve root is affected when it is compressed anteriorly by the bulging or herniated disc and posteriorly against the bony neural arch (Fig. 8). However, there is more than compression to the nerve root pathology in disc protrusion.

It is believed that there are biochemical factors that are toxic to the nerve root when it is significantly compressed. These

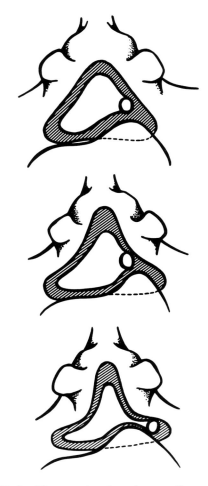

FIG. 8. Diagram to show how a disc protrusion will have different effects depending on the size and shape of the vertebral canal. A protrusion will not significantly compromise a nerve root in a large triangular canal (*top*), nor in a slightly trefoil canal (*middle*). However, a similar disc protrusion into a small, markedly trefoil-shaped canal will significantly compress the nerve root in the lateral recess (*bottom*).

biochemical factors are responsible for root tension signs, particularly limitation of straight leg raising. There are positive and negative risk factors (Table 1).

TABLE 1. *Risk factors for disc protrusion*

Positive risk factors for disc protrusion are:
1. Sedentary work
2. A family history of disc protrusion
3. Smoking
4. An occupation exposed to vibration

Negative risk factors are:
1. Heavy manual work—It is thought that hard work in early life strengthens not only muscles, ligaments, and bones but also the annulus, protecting against disc protrusion.
2. Diabetes—This is a positive risk factor for degenerative change but a negative risk factor for disc protrusion.
3. Isthmic spondylolisthesis when the 5th lumbar vertebra displaces forward, leaving behind a loose neural arch that widens the vertebral canal.
4. Spina bifida occulta, which is associated with a capacious vertebral canal. in the vertebra proximal to the lesion.

Symptoms of disc protrusion are leg pain in a root distribution aggravated by coughing, laughing, and sneezing. Important signs are a trunk list that corrects when lying down (Fig. 9), a positive femoral stretch test (L3 or L4), limited straight leg raising (Fig. 10), and often motor weakness of the extensor digitorum longus. There may be wasting of the extensor digitorum brevis with dermatomal sensory reduction and a reduced knee or ankle reflex.

The natural history of a prolapsed intervertebral disc is generally good. The first pain is usually experienced in the low back, and it may be episodic and severe. With either the first or a later episode, the disc may protrude or herniate further, compromising the nerve root and precipitating symptoms and signs in the leg. The pain is usually so severe that the patient goes to bed for several days. The short-term natural history can take one of several courses. In about 50% of patients, the symptoms and signs will settle down in 1 or 2 wk, resolving completely. In about 20% symptoms will settle slowly over a few weeks but some pain will remain with some limitation of straight leg raising. If symptoms are improving patience is usually rewarded by a good recovery over a few months.

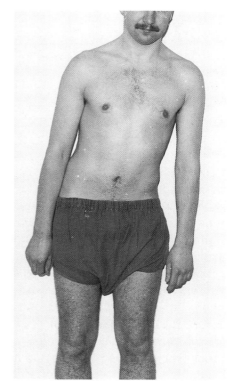

FIG. 9. A patient with a disc protrusion who is listing to the left. The trunk list is abolished by lying down.

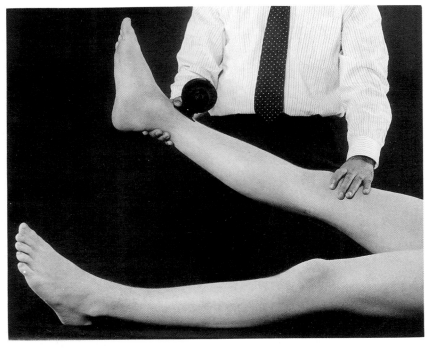

FIG. 10. Limitation of straight leg raising is the most important sign of a disc protrusion.

Approximately 30% of patients, in spite of 2 wk of bed rest, continue to have limited straight leg raising, and these patients are best treated surgically. Without surgery they are likely to continue with a serious disability with sciatic pain, some motor weakness or sensory deficit, and a stiff spine. Without surgery a few may steadily improve over a couple of years, but the majority will be left with a serious back problem for life. A patient with classic root symptoms and signs from disc protrusion who also has bladder symptoms (retention or incontinence), loss of anal tone, and perianal anesthesia has a massive central disc protrusion—a cauda equina syndrome—affecting the sacral roots, requiring emergency surgery. Failure to operate will leave a permanent neurogenic bladder.

Motor weakness or sensory deficit in association with a disc protrusion is not in itself a reason for surgery. However, about 50% of these neurologic changes will remain when the sciatica has resolved and the straight leg raising has improved. Weakness of the big toe or some sensory loss of the outer foot may be a reasonable price to pay for successful conservative management, when one considers the unpredictable risks of surgery.

Straight leg raising that remains limited after 2 wk of bed rest carries a poor prognosis for conservative management.

In particular, when there is a trunk list combined with cross leg pain (pain in the symptomatic leg when lifting the opposite leg), conservative treatment is often unsuccessful. Patients with these three features are best treated with early surgery.

The medium-term prognosis of patients whose first episode of disc protrusion resolves completely with bed rest is variable. Some may remain symptom-free, and others have recurrent episodes until surgery becomes inevitable. Some patients' symptoms partially settle with bed rest, but they continue with a troublesome painful root and, because of chronicity, they require surgery.

The long-term natural history is affected by disc space narrowing. Over a couple of decades after the first symptoms of disc protrusion, the disc space will gradually lose height. The two vertebrae settle together, sometimes with some retrolisthesis. The oblique shape of the apophyseal joints is like tiles on a roof and can cause shingling of the two vertebrae, with posterior displacement of the upper vertebra as the disc space slowly narrows (Fig. 11). If the vertebral canal is trefoil in shape with a deep lateral recess, the posterior displacement of the upper vertebra can compromise the nerve root in the central canal. A rolled ridge of thickened annulus can compress

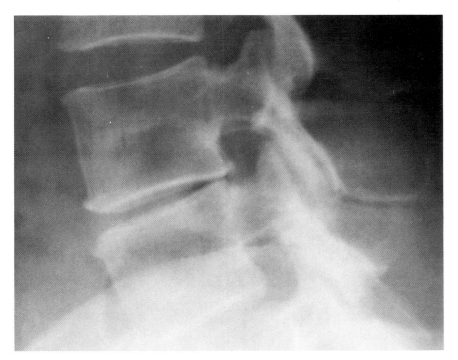

FIG. 11. A lateral radiograph of disc degeneration at L3-4. The upper vertebra has displaced posteriorly, reducing the space in the root canal and foramen.

the root anteriorly against the superior facet posteriorly. In addition, the root canal is composed partly of the vertebra above and partly of the vertebra below and, as the disc loses height, the root canal becomes smaller in cross-sectional area. Both of these abnormalities in the central and in the root canal will limit the available space for the nerve root and be responsible for root entrapment syndrome from lateral canal stenosis. Thus, a patient who makes a successful recovery from disc protrusion in the third decade can experience troublesome root pain again in the fifth or sixth decade from degenerative change.

SPINAL STENOSIS

Spinal stenosis is an anatomic situation that does not always produce symptoms. There are a number of factors

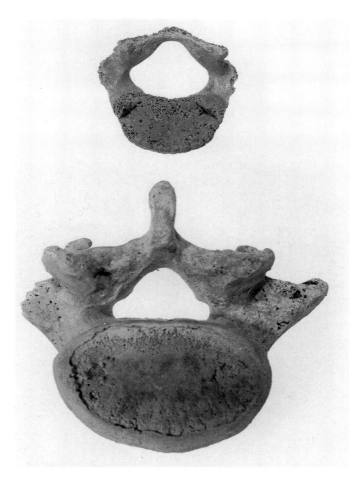

FIG. 12. The vertebral canal area of the 5th lumbar vertebra from a 4-yr-old child is the same as that of the adult.

responsible for stenosis. The first is developmental spinal stenosis. The vertebral canal reaches adult size very early in life. By 4 yr of age, the 5th lumbar vertebral canal has a cross-sectional area the same as in the adult (Fig. 12). The midsagittal diameter is wider than in the adult because of the concave posterior surface of the vertebral body in childhood. The interpedicular diameter gradually widens throughout childhood. The very early maturity of the vertebral canal means that any factors that stunt the canal's growth must act early in life. There are probably environmental factors in utero and early infancy responsible for spinal stenosis; if the canal has not reached satisfactory size by 4 yr of age, there is no opportunity for catch-up growth. Some individuals have spinal stenosis in adult life because of impaired early growth. This can be masked by satisfactory catch-up growth of the long bone, but a development stenosis remains. The midsagittal diameter is the important clinical diameter, but the shape of the canal is as important as its size. Fifteen percent of lumbar vertebral canals are trefoil in shape at L-5 (Figs. 13 and 14). They have a deep lateral recess. The small trefoil canal is an unpleasant combination. Achondroplasia is a rare cause of developmental spinal stenosis.

Second, degenerative spinal stenosis usually contributes to the original developmental narrowing. Degenerative change occurs at the segmental level with the development of a posterior vertebral

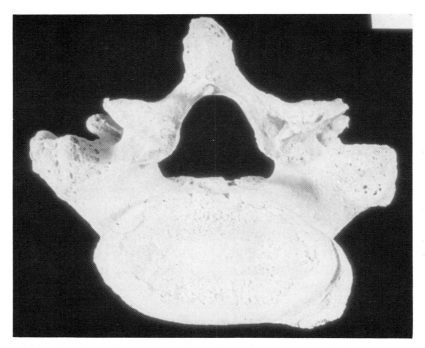

FIG. 13. A 5th lumbar vertebra with a large dome-shaped canal.

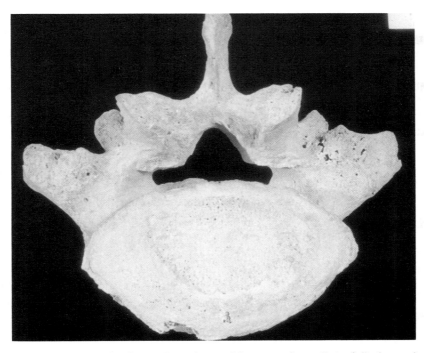

FIG. 14. Fifteen percent of vertebrae have this type of small, trefoil-shaped canal, with a deep lateral recess.

bar adjacent to the disc, a thickened apophyseal joint, osteophytes, a thickened capsule, and a rolled annulus. The ligamentum flavum can lose its elasticity and infold. These degenerative changes can reduce the canal size at each segmental level, and they assume clinical significance if the canal is already developmentally narrow. There are some constitutional causes of spinal degenerative change—diffuse idiopathic spinal hyperostosis (DISH) (Fig. 15) and ossification of the posterior longitudinal ligament, which occurs in Oriental races.

In addition, segmental displacement aggravates the stenosis. Degenerative spondylolisthesis occurs commonly at L4-5 with L-4 vertebra displacing forward on L-5, taking with it an intact neural arch. If the canal is already narrow, this displacement can precipitate symptoms. A degenerative lumbar scoliosis gradually develops in midadult life. Multiple segmental torsional problems can precipitate a stenosis if the canal is already narrow.

Finally, spinal motion dynamically affects the space in the vertebral canal. In flexion the vertebral canal increases in size, and in extension the canal becomes smaller. Canal compromise is aggravated by loss of elasticity in the ligamentum flavum when this ligament buckles into the vertebral canal in exten-

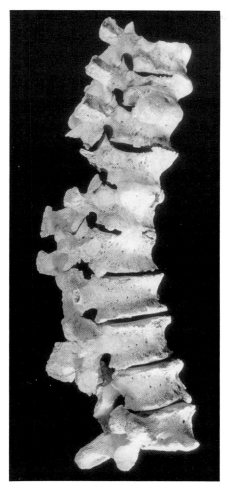

FIG. 15. Vertebrae ankylosed by diffuse idiopathic spinal hyperostosis (DISH). This degenerative change will encroach into the vertebral canal.

sion. The complex motion of walking, when the spine flexes, extends, and rotates, can cause significant compromise if the canal is already narrow.

Clinically, there are two important stenotic syndromes: root entrapment syndrome and neurogenic claudication.

Stenosis is an important factor in the development of these syndromes. The patient with root entrapment syndrome has root pain extending down the leg to the foot, usually severe and constant but without the classic symptoms of disc protrusion. These patients do not have pain aggravated by coughing, laughing, or sneezing. They do not have a trunk list, and they have good straight leg raising. They may not have any abnormal neurologic signs. There may be good reflexes and no motor or sensory dysfunction. However, they do have limited spinal extension because extension further compromises a narrow root canal. The nerve root is tight, either within the root canal in the lateral recess of the central canal or under the superior facet joint (Figs. 16 and 17). It is difficult to understand why the stenosis can have been present for years and the symptoms suddenly develop and why in a majority of patients the symptoms will gradually subside although the stenosis remains. The natural history is encouraging. Most patients without treatment will make a good recovery even if it takes 6 to 12 mo for the symptoms to resolve. Some are helped with an epidural injection. Only about 5% of patients have persistent severe pain that requires surgical decompression.

The second important stenosis syndrome is neurogenic claudication, which can be unilateral or bilateral. There is usually a long history of back pain and a recent history of pain when walking. There is no discomfort in the legs at rest but, after walking a short distance, leg pain increases until, after 100 m or 200

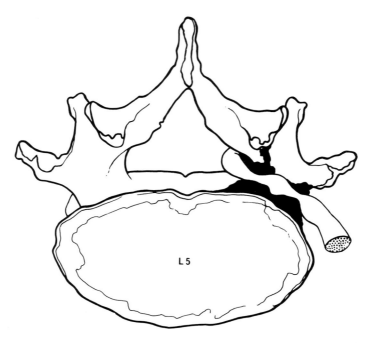

FIG. 16. Diagram to show how degenerative change in the presence of a small root canal can compromise a nerve root.

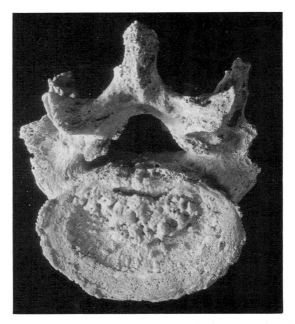

FIG. 17. An osteophyte encroaching into the left root canal at L-5, reducing the space available for the L5 root.

m, the patient will stop and stoop forward. The pathologic condition in patients with bilateral symptoms is usually a two-level central canal stenosis at low pressure around the venous pressure (Figs. 18 and 19). The cauda equina between the two levels of stenosis becomes congested as a result of the venous blockage, and it is believed that the nerve roots then fail to conduct efficiently when the

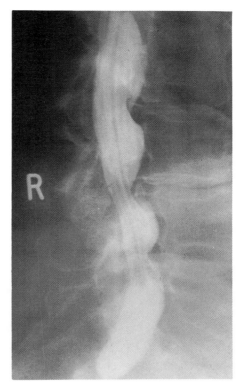

FIG. 19. Myelogram to show the common pattern of multiple level stenosis in a patient with bilateral neurogenic claudication.

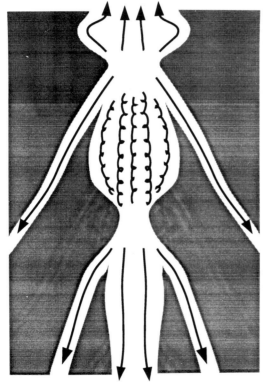

FIG. 18. Diagram to show how a two-level central canal stenosis at around venous pressure will cause venous pooling and congestion of the nerve roots between the two blocks. It is suggested that the nerve roots then fail to conduct effectively when the patient walks.

patient is walking. Fifty percent of these patients with bilateral symptoms have a degenerative spondylolisthesis at L4-5 and a second stenosis at a more proximal level.

In unilateral claudication there is usually a central canal stenosis at one level and a more distal unilateral root canal stenosis causing a two-level venous block of a nerve root (Figs. 20 and 21). Fifty percent of these patients have a degenerative lumbar scoliosis, and the asymmetry of the deformity is responsible for the asymmetric root compression.

Peripheral vascular disease often coexists with spinal stenosis. Men are affected more often than women, and the symptoms are unusual in patients under 50 yr of age.

The natural history of bilateral or unilateral claudication is for patients gradually to reduce their walking distance until they reach a plateau. It is unusual for the symptoms to develop into a serious neuropathy, and patients will not generally go "off their legs." Most are able to continue walking at least 100 m,

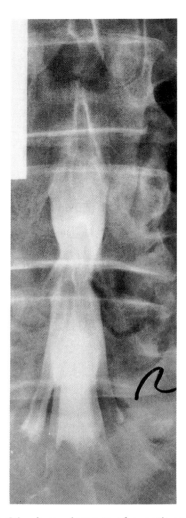

FIG. 21. A myelogram of a patient with right leg claudication and a two-level root stenosis. There is a central canal stenosis at L4-5 and a root stenosis causing a "cutoff" sign of the root at L5-S1.

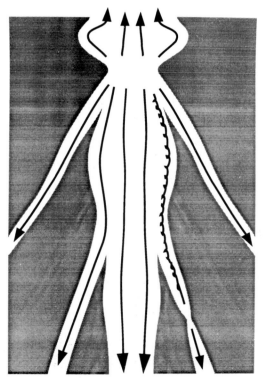

FIG. 20. Diagram to show a congested root as a result of a single-level central canal stenosis and a more distal root canal stenosis. This can be responsible for unilateral claudication.

and many learn to live within this limitation. The severity of symptoms may fluctuate but, once established, the problem remains for life. For the severely disabled, surgical decompression is effective.

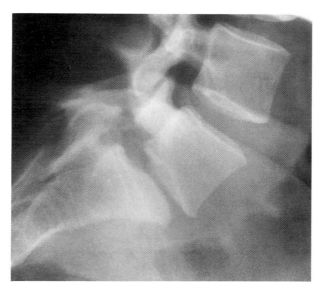

FIG. 22. Lateral radiograph showing an isthmic spondylolisthesis at L-5, with a defect of the neural arch.

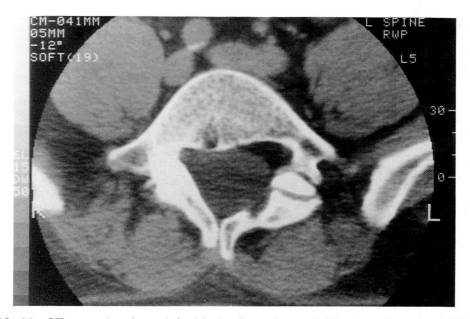

FIG. 23. CT scan showing a left-sided unilateral spondylolysis and a spina bifida occulta. Note the large canal.

ISTHMIC SPONDYLOLISTHESIS

In isthmic spondylolisthesis, there is a defect in the pars interarticularis that may be the result of a stress fracture in childhood, usually at L-5. There is a familial incidence, and it probably occurs in individuals who are predisposed. It occurs bilaterally in approximately 5% of the population (Fig. 22) and unilaterally in about 1% of the population (Fig. 23). The vertebral canal is generally wider than in individuals who do not have a pars defect, and it is unusual for the canal to be trefoil in shape. If there is a defect without any vertebral displacement, it is described as a *spondylolysis* and, if the vertebra displaces forward, leaving behind the neural arch, it is described as a *spondylolisthesis*. The displacement can be up to 30% and is not usually more than 50%. The vertebra does not suddenly slip forward; this is a gradual growth displacement that takes place before puberty. After that time there is generally little change in the degree of displacement. The neurologic tissues have adapted to this change in shape.

Isthmic spondylolisthesis may cause no symptoms at all. When it is responsible for pain, it is usually low back pain, sometimes referred around the pelvis or into the thighs. It may cause root pain with root entrapment due to the degenerative change around the defect. Patients with isthmic spondylolisthesis are less likely to present with disc protrusion than are the rest of the population and are less likely to have neurogenic claudication because the vertebral canal is relatively large (Fig. 24). Isthmic spondylolisthesis at L-4 follows a stress frac-

ture in adult life, usually in sportsmen and women.

When symptoms of backache first present in an adolescent with an isthmic spondylolisthesis, the natural history is a little uncertain. Many surgeons recommend fusion, which is usually very successful and will permit normal activity at work and in sports. However, the natural history has not been carefully assessed with a randomized trial, and some young patients with an acute episode of back pain associated with a spondylolisthesis do have a natural resolution of symptoms if left alone.

When a patient of any age first presents with acute back pain and a spondylolisthesis, it is important to determine whether there is a new stress fracture. Technetium-99 bone scanning is helpful and, if positive, a period of immobilization can result in sound union and relief of symptoms.

However, many patients after the first symptoms of back pain from spondylolisthesis have the beginning of a chronic problem. It may vary in degree but usually continues for years as a source of back pain that limits activity. In older life, however, the degenerative change associated with a spondylolisthesis at L-5 will result in a degree of stabilization and a "self-fusion" (Fig. 25). The prognosis of L-4 isthmic spondylolisthesis is not good, and if painful it is probably best treated by fusion (Fig. 26).

When root entrapment syndrome is associated with isthmic spondylolisthesis, in some patients the symptoms will settle and in others the pain will steadily increase, requiring surgery (Fig. 27). It is not possible to discriminate between

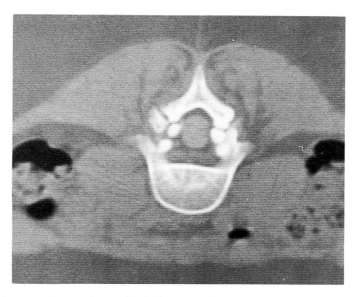

FIG. 24. CT scan of a patient with isthmic spondylolisthesis at L-5, showing the large vertebral canal. Symptomatic disc protrusion or neurogenic claudication would be unusual.

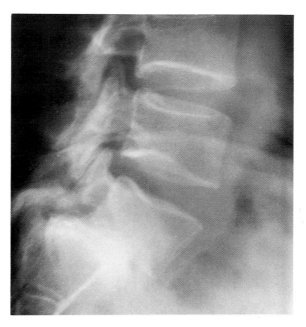

FIG. 25. A marked spondylolisthesis at L5-S1, which has stabilized with degenerative change.

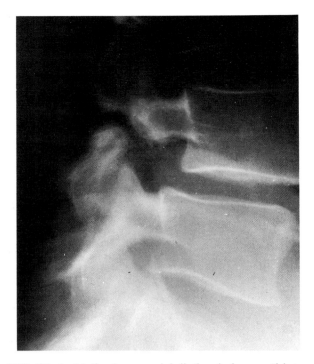

FIG. 26. L-4 isthmic spondylolisthesis in an athlete.

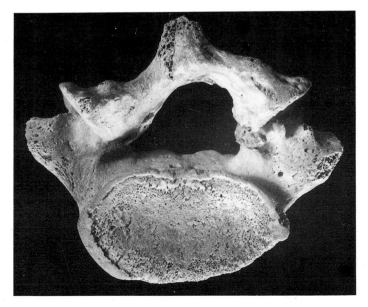

FIG. 27. A unilateral spondylolysis. The hypertrophic bone at the site of the defect can disturb the L5 nerve root at this site.

these two groups without waiting some time to observe the natural history.

DYSPLASTIC SPONDYLOLISTHESIS

Dysplastic spondylolisthesis is a failure of development of the neural arch. The apophyseal joints are small and dysplastic, and the pars is thin and attenuated. There may or may not be defects in the pars, and there may or may not be a spina bifida occulta. The displacement is usually much greater in the dysplastic spondylolisthesis than in the isthmic variety, with more than 50% vertebral displacement. The anterior part of the upper surface of the sacrum becomes convex as the L-5 vertebra displaces and rotates forward on the front of the first piece of the sacrum. Sometimes the L-5 vertebral body is almost totally dislocated before the patient presents. The symptoms are deformity and back pain varying in degree. A crisis can develop in the adolescent, with acute pain and hamstring spasm requiring surgical fusion. Reduction before fusion is proposed by some but is illogical if one believes that the deformity is a growth phenomenon. The neurologic tissues have adapted to growth, and great care must be exercised when attempting to reduce a severely displaced spondylolisthesis lest neurologic damage occurs.

DEGENERATIVE SPONDYLOLISTHESIS

This generally occurs at L4-5 and more often in women who are over 50 yr old. It can produce three distinct syndromes.

The first is chronic low back pain; once established, pain tends to persist. Second, it can be responsible for root entrapment syndrome. The displacement is not marked but, as it slowly develops in the postmenopausal period, root entrapment can steadily get worse and be very disabling. Surgical decompression and fusion is usually indicated. Third, some patients will experience bilateral neurogenic claudication if there is a more proximal secondary stenosis.

SPINAL FRACTURE

Wedge compression fracture, the most common vertebral fracture, occurs when the anterior part of the vertebral body is compressed into a wedge. This is usually the result of a fall from a height when the momentum flexes the trunk forward, compressing the anterior aspect of one or several vertebral bodies. It is sometimes associated with fractures of the heel bones and sometimes with a fracture of the base of the skull. The back is usually painful and tender at the site of the fracture. Depending on the degree of compression, the spinous process is prominent, causing a gibbus or a kyphosis.

Osteoporotic wedge compression fractures of the thoracic spine occur mainly in osteoporotic elderly women, with an incidence of about 15 new fractures per 1,000 person-years in women over 50 yr of age. There is low bone mineral density with a deficiency in bone mass per unit volume. The bone present is essentially normal, but the mass is reduced. The mass is reduced physiologically with age at

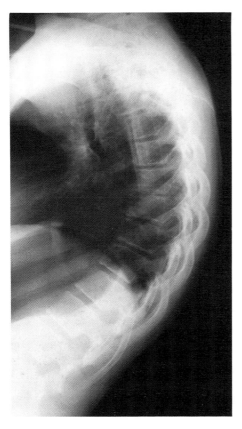

FIG. 28. Thoracic kyphosis from multiple minor compression fractures in an osteoporotic elderly woman.

about 1% per annum after the menopause, but it can be reduced also by immobilization, corticosteroid drugs, and metabolic disorders. One or several vertebral bodies may collapse either slowly or suddenly, giving spontaneous severe back pain that usually resolves over a few weeks. The resultant kyphosis is a cosmetic problem (Fig. 28) but not necessarily a functional disability. Pathologic fracture must be excluded.

Burst fracture is a comminuted fracture of the vertebral body, involving both the anterior and the posterior cortex, after an axial load without flexion. The vertebral body bursts out in several directions as the disc fractures the vertebral endplate (Figs. 29 and 30). Fracture of the neural arch follows flexion, rotation, or shear injury (Fig. 31).

There are three important questions to be asked when considering vertebral fractures. The first is whether back pain will be temporary or permanent. Fractures of the spine will unite like any other bony injury, and pain is usually temporary. A few individuals, however, do develop chronic back pain as a result of altered spinal mechanics. The physiologic lumbar lordosis is important for the spine's strength and, if this arch is lost as a result of a wedge fracture, the spine can be permanently weakened. For the majority, however, the fractured spine can be compatible with a pain-free, normally functioning back.

The second question is whether as a result of fracture the spine is stable or unstable. Instability means that the spine is able to move in an excessive or erratic manner at the level of the fracture. This can then damage the spinal cord above L-2 or the cauda equina if the fracture is in the lower lumbar region. A patient whose spine is unstable after a fracture is at risk of neurologic damage and must be treated either by very careful nursing or preferably by surgical fixation.

Stability can be assessed by the severity of the fracture. We think of the spine as three columns. The anterior column comprises the anterior cortex of the ver-

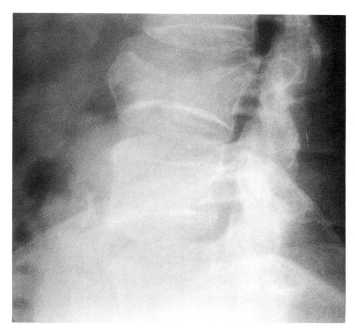

FIG. 29. Lateral radiograph of a 28-yr-old man who fell from a height. There is a burst fracture of L-2 affecting the anterior and posterior cortex of the vertebral body. A CT scan is required to exclude a neural arch fracture, which would cause spinal instability.

tebral bodies and the anterior part of the discs, the middle column comprises the posterior cortex of the vertebral bodies and the posterior part of the discs, and the posterior column comprises the neural arch and the posterior ligaments. If one of these columns is intact, the spine is probably stable. In other words, it is possible to have a burst fracture affecting the anterior and posterior cortex of the vertebral bodies with a stable spine because the neural arch is intact. It is not easy to identify the severity of the bony injury on plain radiographs and, if instability is suspected, a computed tomographic (CT) scan is the imaging method of choice.

It is unusual for a fracture of the thoracic spine to be unstable if the ribs and sternum are intact. However, when a patient has a fractured sternum or fractured ribs in association with tenderness of the thoracic spine, an unstable spinal fracture should be assumed until proved otherwise. Such a patient should be nursed with extreme care before imaging.

Any patient admitted with a neck injury or any patient admitted unconscious after trauma should be given a cervical collar and assumed to have an unstable neck injury until proved otherwise.

The third question is whether the fracture is associated with neurologic symptoms or

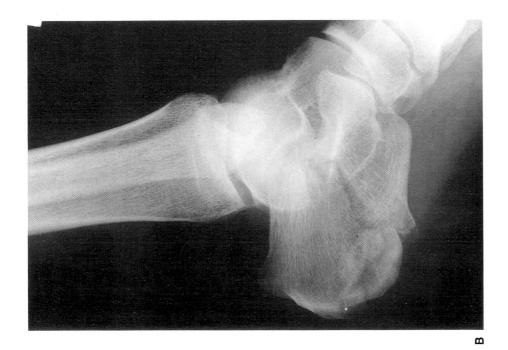

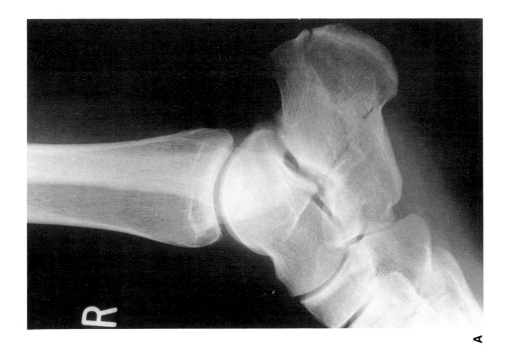

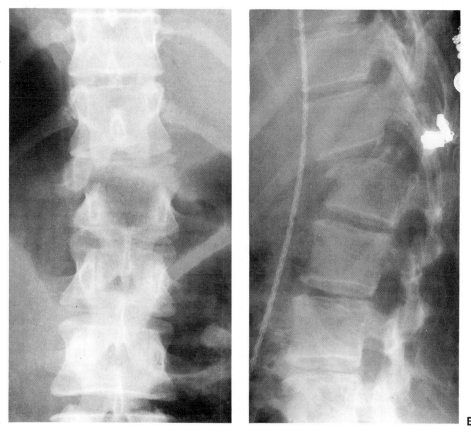

A   B

FIG. 31. AP and lateral radiographs of a 32-yr-old woman who had a head-on collision in her car. She was wearing a lap belt and sustained a flexion shearing injury. She had a complete paraplegia at T12-L1.

FIG. 30. The same patient fractured both os calces, always to be considered with a burst fracture of the spine.

signs. There may be a complete spinal cord lesion from either transection of the cord or contusion. This constitutes an emergency because early reduction of a dislocated neck with cord contusion can result in full neurologic recovery. In the thoracic and lumbar spine, it is unusual for a complete neurologic lesion to recover with surgical decompression. A partial neurologic injury, however, can recover with prompt surgical decompression. Increasing neurologic compromise can result from extradural bleeding or thrombosis after trauma.

Thus, the optimum treatment for an unstable spine and a spinal fracture associated with a partial neurologic disc function is surgical stabilization and/or decompression.

SUGGESTED READING

1. Bohlman HH. Current concepts review: treatment of fractures and dislocations of the thoracic and lumbar spine. *J Bone Joint Surg [Am]* 1985;67A:165–169.
2. Cooper C, Melton LJ. Vertebral fractures. *Br Med J* 1992;304:793–794.
3. Hardcastle P, Annear P, Foster DH, Chakera TM, McCormick C, Khagure M, Burnett A. Spinal abnormalities in young fast bowlers. *J Bone Joint Surg [Br]*1992;74B:421–425.
4. Khuffash B, Porter RW. Cross leg pain and trunk list. *Spine* 1989;14:602–603.
5. Mumford J, Weinstein JN, Spratt KF, Goel VK. Thoracolumbar burst fractures: the clinical efficacy and outcome of nonoperative management. AcroMed Award Paper. *Spine* 1993;18(8): 955–970.
6. Porter RW. *Management of back pain.* 2nd ed. New York: Churchill Livingstone; 1993.
7. Porter RW, Ward D. Cauda equina dysfunction: the significance of multiple level pathology. *Spine* 1992;17:9–15.
8. Porter RW, Wicks M, Hibbert C. The size of the lumbar spinal canal in the symptomatology of disc lesions. *J Bone Joint Surg [Br]* 1978;60B:485–487.
9. Urban J, Maroudas A. The chemistry of the intervertebral disc in relation to its physiological function and requirements. *Clin Rheum Dis* 1980;6(1):51–57.

4

Understanding the Accuracy of Diagnostic Tests

Richard A. Deyo

Departments of Medicine and Health Services, University of Washington,
Seattle, Washington 98105, USA

Key Points

- Diagnosis is an inherently difficult exercise.

- The history, physical examination, and diagnostic tests affect the probability of making an accurate diagnosis.

- The prevalence of true causes of back pain must be distinguished from the prevalence of positive anatomic studies.

- A herniated disc is seen in 20% to 40% of CT, myelogram, and magnetic resonance imaging (MRI) studies among normal persons.

- For clinical decision-making purposes, false-positive imaging tests are very common, although anatomic findings are probably real.

- Sensitivity is the proportion of persons with the disease who have a positive test (PID—positive in disease).

- Specificity is the ability of a test correctly to identify patients without disease (NIH—negative in health).

Back pain can be a symptom of many widely divergent diseases. However, it has been estimated that up to 85% of patients cannot be given a definitive diagnosis because of the weak associations among symptoms, pathologic changes, and imaging results. In many instances, we assume that these undiagnosed cases are a result of musculoligamentous injury or degenerative changes in the spine.

Many of these episodes of back pain respond to symptomatic and physical measures.

However, some causes of back pain are surgically remediable, and some are due to systemic diseases, such as cancer or disseminated infection, that require specific therapy. Thus, careful diagnostic evaluation is important.

THE PREVALENCE OF SPINAL DISEASES CAUSING LOW BACK PAIN

As we shall see, the prevalence of disease in the population under consideration is critical to interpreting diagnostic tests. The predictive value of a test (defined below) is highly dependent on the prevalence of target diseases in the population being studied. Table 1 shows estimates of the prevalence of various diseases among patients with low back pain seen in primary care. National survey data demonstrate that the prevalence of serious specific diseases is higher in specialty practices such as orthopaedic surgery or neurosurgery, so that these figures must be modified according to the referral filters through which one's own patients pass.

The prevalence of these conditions as true causes of back pain should be distinguished from their prevalence in

TABLE 1. *The prevalence of spinal diseases causing low back pain (LBP) and selected features of the medical history*

Condition	Estimated prevalence in primary care patients with LBP	Other common historical findings
Nonspecific low back pain (often attributed to lumbar strain or osteoarthritis)	0.85	All ages affected
Vertebral compression fracture	0.04	Falls, trauma, corticosteroid use; most common in postmenopausal white women
Spondylolisthesis	0.03	May be asymptomatic; sometimes sciatica or pseudoclaudication
Herniated intervertebral disc	0.02[a]	Sciatica in 95% of those requiring surgery; peak incidence age 30–55.
Spinal stenosis	?	Pseudoclaudication; peak incidence over age 50
Spinal malignancy (primary or metastatic)	0.007	Age >50, weight loss, lymphadenopathy; breast, prostate, and lung are common primaries.
Ankylosing spondylitis	0.003	Morning stiffness, improves with exercise, long duration, most common in men under age 40
Infection (epidural abscess, osteomyelitis, disc space infection)	0.0001	i.v.[b] drug abuse, UTI[b] urinary catheters, skin infection, unexplained fever

[a] Estimated prevalence of herniated discs requiring surgery; anatomic evidence of herniated disc is more common, even in asymptomatic persons (20–30%)

[b] i.v., intravenous; UTI, urinary tract infection.

anatomic studies. Thus, for example, anatomic evidence of a herniated disc is found in 20% to 30% of CT and MRI studies among normal persons. However, these seem to be asymptomatic herniations that cause no clinical disease. It seems that the proportion of all persons with low back pain who eventually undergo disc surgery is only about 2%. Thus, for clinical decision-making purposes, "false-positive" test results are very common, although the anatomic findings are probably real.

Because identifying a definitive diagnosis may often be impossible for the patient with low back pain, the early diagnostic evaluation can reasonably focus on three basic questions: Is there a serious systemic disease causing the pain? Is there neurologic compromise? Is there social or psychologic distress that may amplify or prolong pain?

FINDING THE ACCURACY OF A DIAGNOSTIC TEST: SOME DEFINITIONS

Understanding the accuracy of any diagnostic test, whether it is part of the physical examination or an expensive imaging procedure, presumes that we can know the ultimate truth about a patient. Thus, some "gold standard" for the diagnosis is required. Typically, the gold standard is a definitive diagnosis attained by biopsy, surgery, autopsy, long-term follow-up, or some superior diagnostic test. Unfortunately, none of these gold standards are themselves infallible, but we must assume that there is some gold standard that is reasonably acceptable.

An even thornier problem for the study of back pain is that many commonly used diagnoses do not have widely agreed-upon definitions or criteria. Thus, clinical diagnoses of sacroiliac disorders, fibrositis, disc degeneration, facet joint syndrome, spine instability, and trigger point syndromes as causes of back pain remain controversial. Many of these diagnoses, like coccydynia in an earlier era, may ultimately prove to be little more than medical fads and fashions. For example, recent studies cast doubt on the ability of multiple observers to agree on the existence of physical findings such as trigger points and sacroiliac joint dysfunction. Recent randomized trials for facet joint pain and trigger points have been negative, challenging the notion that we can reliably diagnose or treat such conditions. Where such ambiguity exists, detailed patient descriptions may be preferable to poorly defined diagnostic labels.

Assuming that we have an acceptable gold standard, the next question is how a given maneuver on the physical examination or a diagnostic test compares with the results of the gold standard. In judging test efficacy we hope to find data from an independent, blinded comparison of the diagnostic test with the gold standard result. Often this comparison will result in statistics such as the sensitivity and specificity of a diagnostic test, but this jargon is often misunderstood.

In its simplest form, evaluation of a diagnostic test requires the creation of a 2 x 2 table such as that shown in Table 2. If the critical reader cannot identify or construct such a table from an article about a diagnostic test, he or she should be suspicious about whether the terms

TABLE 2. *The typical 2x2 table for comparing a diagnostic test to a "gold standard"*

Result	Gold standard		Total
	Patient has the disease	Patient does not have the disease	
Diagnostic test result			
Positive	(*a*)true positives	(*b*)false positives	*a+b*
Negative	(*c*) false negatives	(*d*) true negatives	*c+d*
Total	*a+c*	*b+d*	*a+b+c+d*
Stable properties			
Sensitivity = $a/(a+c)$			
Specificity = $d/(b+d)$			
Frequency or prevalence-dependent properties			
Predictive value of a positive test $a/(a+b)$			
Predictive value of a negative test $d/(c+d)$			
Prevalence of disease in the sample: $(a+c)/(a+b+c+d)$			

have been used correctly and whether the test has been appropriately evaluated. In Table 2, there are a total of $(a+c)$ patients who have the disease under consideration, and *a* patients had a positive test result. Those in Category *c* truly have the disease but had a false-negative test. The sensitivity of the test is defined as $a/(a+c)$ and is often expressed as a percentage. This indicates the proportion of persons with a disease who have a positive test, and the acronym PID (positive in disease) has been coined to help remember the definition of sensitivity (although you may have learned a different definition of the acronym from the gynecologists).

To be clinically useful, a test must not only be positive when the disease is present, but also be negative when the disease is absent. The ability of a test to identify patients without disease correctly is called *specificity* and is calculated in Table 2 as $d/(d+b)$. In this case, patients in Category *d* have true negative results, while those in Category *b* have no disease but have false-positive test results. The acronym NIH

(negative in health) may help to remember this definition, even though you may have thought that the acronym stood for National Institutes of Health.

The sensitivity and specificity of a test are sometimes called *vertical properties* because they are calculated using the vertical columns in Table 2. It can be shown that these characteristics actually vary somewhat according to the severity of disease being evaluated, but it is a common generalization to assume that these are stable properties of a test.

Sensitivity and specificity are useful characteristics but do not reflect how test results are used in clinical practice. In reality, we do not have the results of a gold standard to go by, or we would not be doing the less definitive diagnostic test. In fact, we are less interested in knowing how likely the test is to be positive when the patient has disease than in the likelihood that the patient has the disease given a positive test result. This probability is obtained by working horizontally in the table, rather than vertically, and is known as the *predictive value* of a test result. The predictive value asks, "Given a positive test result, how likely is it to be a true positive?" The positive predictive value of a test is shown in Table 2 by the value $a/(a+b)$. The predictive value of a negative test is similarly represented by $d/(c+d)$.

In contrast to sensitivity and specificity, which are at least theoretically stable, predictive values can vary dramatically according to the prevalence of disease (also known as *prior probability*) among patients who receive the test. The prevalence of disease in the patients shown in Table 2 is simply $(a+c)/(a+b+c+d)$.

Table 3 illustrates widely differing predictive values depending on the likelihood of disease in a population under study. In the top half of the table, 60% of the patients who receive an MRI scan

actually have a herniated disc. This would be typical of the probability in a patient with sciatica, positive straight leg raising, and a poor response to conservative therapy. In this circumstance, the predictive value of a positive test is 87%. However, among unselected patients with back pain alone, the probability of disease is very different. For example, in primary care practices, only about 3% of patients with back complaints have herniated disc as a cause of pain. If MRI were used for every patient in this circumstance, even though sensitivity and specificity remain the same, the predictive value of a positive test would be only 12%. Thus, even with a positive test result, the patient's true cause of pain would more likely be something other than the herniated disc identified by the imaging test. This is why

TABLE 3. *Effects of disease prevalence on predictive value of a diagnostic test*

Test result	True state of reality— patient symptoms are due to		Total
	Herniated disc	Other condition	
Sciatica			
MRI positive	540	80	620
MRI negative	60	320	380
Total	600	400	1000
Predictive value of a positive test 540/620=0.87			
Lumbar back pain alone			
MRI positive	27	194	221
MRI negative	3	776	779
Total	30	970	1000
Predictive value of a positive test 27/221=0.12			

This example compares a test for herniated disc among patients with sciatica versus patients with back pain alone. We assumed test sensitivity of 90% and specificity of 80% (roughly the characteristics of MRI for this diagnosis). We estimated the prevalence of herniated discs as the cause of pain in patients with sciatica to be 60% and among those without sciatica to be 3%. Of patients with sciatica, 60% have a herniated disc, so for 1,000 hypothetical patients the results should be as shown at the top. We estimate that 3% of patients seen for lumbar back pain alone have a herniated disc, so for 1,000 hypothetical patients the results should be as shown at the bottom.
From Deyo et al. (1994).

diagnostic tests can be so misleading when they are applied to patients who are unlikely to have the target condition to begin with. This is also why most thoughtful observers insist that patients have appropriate clinical findings, such as sciatica and nerve root tension signs, before ever requesting an imaging test for herniated discs.

Understanding the definitions of these statistics for test accuracy can help to understand when a test is good for ruling in or ruling out a disease. When the specificity of a test is extremely high, a positive test result can help "rule in" the target disease. The acronym SpPin has been coined to help remember this situation. In contrast, an extremely sensitive diagnostic test is more helpful for ruling out a disease. When a highly sensitive test is negative, the likelihood of disease becomes extremely small. Thus, when the sensitivity from a test is high, a negative response rules out the target disease, resulting in the acronym SnNout.

Although there are many potential sources of bias in studies evaluating diagnostic tests, we have pointed out the rudiments of such investigation. Those who wish to learn more about critically evaluating studies of diagnostic tests can find further details elsewhere. Remember that many diagnostic tests produce more complex results than simply positive or negative findings. That is, like many blood tests, they may produce quantitative results with a wide range of answers and a wide range of potential sensitivities and specificities depending on the cutoff selected to represent an abnormal test result. Other techniques have been developed for quantifying and describing test accuracy in this circumstance (e.g., receiver operating characteristic or ROC curves), but a discussion of these techniques is beyond the scope of this chapter. Again, excellent sources are available elsewhere.

THE ACCURACY OF THE HISTORY AND PHYSICAL EXAMINATION

Table 4 provides estimates of the accuracy of the medical history in diagnosing several spine diseases that cause low back pain. This table shows, for example, that the clinical history can be extremely valuable in helping to rule in or rule out cancer as the cause of back pain. For example, a previous history of cancer has such high specificity (0.98) that such patients should be considered to have cancer until proven otherwise. However, the sensitivity of this finding is rather low. Since most cancer patients report that their back pain is unrelieved by bed rest, this is a highly sensitive finding and helps to rule out metastatic cancer. It is so nonspecific, however, that a positive result helps only modestly to raise the likelihood of disease. Combinations of historical findings can virtually exclude cancer as the cause of back pain. For example, in a study of almost 2,000 patients with back pain in a walk-in clinic, no cancer was identified among patients under age 50 without a history of cancer, unexplained weight loss, or failure of conservative therapy (combined sensitivity of 100%).

The accuracy of the history for detecting spinal osteomyelitis is less clear and

TABLE 4. *Estimated accuracy of the medical history in the diagnosis of spine diseases causing low back pain*

Disease to be detected	Reference	Medical history	Sensitivity	Specificity[a]
Cancer	15	Age . 50 yr	0.77	0.71
		Previous history of cancer	0.31	0.98
		Unexplained weignt loss	0.15	0.94
		Failure to improve with a month of therapy	0.31	0.90
		No relief with bed rest	0.90	0.46
		Duration of pain >1 mo	0.50	0.81
		Age . 50 yr *or* history of cancer *or* unexplained weight loss *or* failure of conservative therapy	1.00	0.60
Spinal osteomyelitis	29	Intravenous drug abuse, urinary tract infection. or skin infection	0.40	N A
Compression fracture	Unpublished data[b]	Age . 50 yr	0.84	0.61
		Age . 70 yr	0.22	0.96
		Trauma	0.30	0.85
		Corticosteroid use	0.06	0.995
Herniated disc	18, 30	Sciatica	0.95	0.88
Spinal stenosis	31	Pseudoclaudication	0.60	N A
		Age . 50 yr	0.90[c]	0.70
Ankylosing Spondylitis	16	4 out of 5 positive responses[d]	0.23	0.82
		Age at onset . 40 yr	1.00	0.07
		Pain not relieved supine	0.80	0.49
		Morning back stiffness	0.64	0.59
		Pain duration . 3 mo	0.71	0.54

From Deyo et al. (1992).

[a] NA indicates not available.

[b] From 833 patients with back pain at a walk-in clinic, all of whom received plain lumbar roentgenograms.

[c] Author's estimate.

[d] The five screening questions: (1)Onset of back discomfort before age 40 years? (2)Did the problem begin slowly? (3)Persistence for at least 3 months? (4)Morning stiffness? (5)Improved by exercise?

is probably disappointing. The physical examination is helpful here, however, because fever is relatively specific (0.98) and spine tenderness to percussion is relatively sensitive (0.86).

Similarly, the history is valuable in identifying patients with possible compression fractures. Because most compression fractures are a result of generalized osteoporosis, they often lack a history of trauma. Nonetheless, trauma is a relatively specific finding and should always be questioned. Patients on long-term corticosteroid therapy should be considered to have a compression fracture until proven otherwise. Similarly, age over 70 yr is a relatively specific finding, and compression fractures should always be considered in this population.

Ankylosing spondylitis is a very rare disease, and the clinical evaluation is only moderately accurate. Thus, in practice, this diagnosis is usually suspected only after back pain is persistent and an x-ray film is obtained. Table 4 shows the accuracy of some historical questions for ankylosing spondylitis. Perhaps the most useful of these historical findings is the age of onset. If back pain did not begin before age 40, ankylosing spondylitis becomes very unlikely.

Because ankylosing spondylitis results in fusion of adjacent vertebrae, tests of spine mobility have been advocated for helping to make this diagnosis. Unfortunately, reduced spine flexion is not specific for inflammatory spondyloarthopathies and is equally common in patients with chronic back pain or spine tumors. Reduced chest expansion, using a strict criterion such as less than 2.5 cm as abnormal, is very specific but is insensitive in detecting early ankylosing spondylitis.

Finally, tests for sacroiliac joint tenderness such as hip extension, anteroposterior pelvic pressure, lateral pelvic compression, and direct pressure on the sacroiliac joints have been advocated to distinguish ankylosing spondylitis from mechanical spine conditions. However, these tests are poorly reproducible among examiners and relatively inaccurate in distinguishing ankylosing spondylitis from mechanical disorders.

Identifying Neurologic Compromise

Lumbar spine disorders may produce neurologic abnormalities in the lower extremities. Most commonly, these are caused by herniated intervertebral discs, but they are occasionally a result of spinal stenosis, infections, or cancer.

The first indication of possible nerve root irritation is usually a history suggesting sciatica. Typically, true radiculopathy produces pain radiating below the knee (usually to the foot or ankle) and is associated with numbness or paresthesia. The pain is often aggravated by coughing, sneezing, or a Valsalva maneuver.

The absence of sciatica (or femoral nerve radicular pain) makes a clinically important disc herniation very unlikely. That is, it is such a sensitive finding (about 0.95) that its absence almost rules out a clinically important disc herniation.

A true radiculopathy is further suggested by nerve root tension signs. For the sciatic nerve, this generally means straight leg raising; for the femoral nerve, however, this means the femoral nerve stretch test (flexing the knee with the patient prone). If we define a positive straight leg raising test as one that reproduces the patient's sciatica at less than 60° of leg elevation, we can estimate the sensitivity and specificity of this test for lumbar disc herniations. Table 5 suggests that straight leg raising is moderately sensitive but relatively nonspecific in the diagnosis of a herniated disc.

Crossed straight leg raising occurs when straight leg raising is performed on the patient's well leg and elicits pain in the leg with sciatica. This test is substantially less sensitive than is ipsilateral straight leg raising but, as shown in Table 5, it is substantially more specific. Thus, it is more effective as a "rule-in" test, whereas ipsilateral straight leg raising is more effective as a rule-out test.

TABLE 5. *Estimated accuracy of physical examination for lumbar disc herniation among patients with sciatica*

Test	Source	Sensitivity[a]	Specificity[a]	Comments
Ipsilateral straight leg raising	13,18	0.80	0.40	Positive test result: leg pain at <60°
Crossed straight leg raising	13,30	0.25	0.90	Positive test result: reproduction of contralateral pain
Ankle dorsiflexion weakness	13,30	0.35	0.70	HNP[b] usually at L4-5 (80%)
Great toe extensor (60%) weakness	13,17	0.50	0.70	HNP usually at L5-S 1 or L4-5 (30%)
Impaired ankle reflex	13,30	0.50	0.60	HNP usually at L5-SI; absent reflex increases specificity
Sensory loss	17,18	0.50	0.50	Area of loss poor predictor of HNP level
Patella reflex	1	0.50	...	For upper lumbar HNP only
Ankle plantar flexion weakness	13	0.06	0.95	
Quadriceps weakness	13	0.01	0.99	

[a] Sensitivity and specificity were calculated by the authors of the present report. Values represent rounded averages where multiple references were available. All results are from surgical case series.
[b] HNP, herniated nucleus pulposus.
From Deyo et al. (1992).

Since almost 98% of clinically important lumbar disc herniations occur at the L4-5 or L5-S1 levels, the most common neurologic impairments are those of the L5 and S1 nerve roots. Thus, by far the most common neurologic impairments are weakness of ankle and great toe dorsiflexors (L5), reduced ankle reflexes (S1), and sensory deficits in the feet (L5 and S1). Table 5 shows the approximate sensitivity and specificity of each of these physical findings, which are only modest in most cases.

However, a combination of tests is sometimes better able to rule in or rule out a herniated disc. For example, almost 90% of patients with surgically proven disc herniations have either impaired ankle reflexes or weak foot dorsiflexion (combined sensitivity = 0.90). Thus, the absence of both findings helps to rule out a herniated disc as a cause of the patient's pain. Similarly, the greater the number of positive findings related to straight leg raising or neurologic examination, the greater the likelihood of a herniated disc being found at surgery (the higher specificity becomes).

A far less common neurologic syndrome than simple radiculopathy is the cauda equina syndrome. Occasionally, a massive midline disc herniation may compress the entire cauda equina, resulting in bowel or bladder dysfunction and bilateral lower extremity signs. Fortunately, the cauda equina syndrome has been reported in only 1% to 2% of all patients who undergo lumbar disc surgery. The most consistent finding in these patients is urinary retention, with a sensitivity of about 90%. Unilateral or bilateral sciatica, sensory and motor deficits, and abnormal straight leg raising are all common in this condition, with sensitivities of 80% or more. Sensory deficits in a saddle distribution have a sensitivity of about 75%, and anal sphincter tone is diminished in 60% to 80% of cases. The specificity of these findings is unknown.

These data on the clinical evaluation suggest that x-ray films and other imaging tests are not necessary for every patient with low back pain. Indeed, because there is a substantial risk of misleading results and because variability in interpretation is common, many observers suggest highly selective use of imaging tests. The Quebec Task Force on Spinal Disorders recommended plain x-ray films only in the face of neurologic deficits, age over 50 or under 20 yr, or the presence of fever, trauma, or findings suggestive of cancer. As shown in Table 4, negative answers to several screening questions can help to almost exclude malignancy on the basis of history alone.

As we will argue below, magnetic resonance imaging and computed tomography can be used even more selectively, usually for surgical planning. Because abnormal findings are extremely common in asymptomatic persons, valid interpretation of these imaging tests always requires correlation with the history and physical examination.

THE ACCURACY OF COMMON IMAGING TESTS

As previously noted, clinically irrelevant findings are common for both plain x-ray films and more sophisticated lumbar imaging tests. Table 6 shows a list of plain x-ray findings that are probably irrelevant, based on large epidemiologic studies of asymptomatic persons. Similarly, Table 7 shows the high prevalence of several abnormalities in normal volunteers on CT and MRI images. The findings demonstrated in Table 7 seem to represent true anatomic abnormalities, and yet they are clinically irrelevant. Thus, for decision-making purposes, they can be regarded as false-positive results, and these greatly reduce the specificity of these spine-imaging tests.

TABLE 6. *Radiologic abnormalities in the lumbar spine with significance for low back pain*

Classification	Abnormality
Irrelevant	Single disc narrowing and spondylosis
	Facet arthrosis, subluxation, and tropism
	Disc calcification
	Lumbarization, sacralization
	Intraspongy disc herniation (Schmorl's nodes)
	Spina bifida occulta
	Accessory ossicles
	Mild-moderate scoliosis
Questionable	Spondylolysis
	Retrolisthesis
	Severe lumbar scoliosis (>80°)
	Severe lordosis
Definite	Spondylolisthesis
	Lumbar osteochondrosis (Scheuermann)
	Congenital/traumatic kyphosis
	Osteoporosis
	Marked multiple disc narrowing
	Ankylosing spondylitis

From Nachemson (1976).

TABLE 7. *Computed tomography and magnetic resonance imaging results on normal subjects*

CT results: "normal subjects" (N = 52)

	Age	
	Under 40	Over 40
Herniated disc	20%	27%
Spinal stenosis	0%	3%
Facet abnormality	0%	10%
Any abnormality	20%	50%

From Wiesel et al. (1984).

MRI results: "normal" subjects (N = 67)

	Age	
	Under 60	Over 60
Herniated disc	22%	36%
Spinal stenosis	1%	21%
Bulging disc	54%	79%
Degenerated disc	46%	93%

From Boden et al. (1990).

Table 8 summarizes several studies of the sensitivity and specificity of various tests for the diagnosis of herniated lumbar discs. In several cases the tabled estimates of sensitivity and specificity are synthetic, informally integrating data from several studies. For illustrative purposes, the table also shows the predictive values of these tests for patients with a high prior probability of disease and for a patient population with a low prior probability of disease. These data emphasize that these tests are far from perfect and remind us that diagnosis is inherently a probabilistic exercise. In particular, the predictive value of a positive test among patients with a low clinical probability is very disappointing and likely to be misleading. In a patient without appropriate history and physical findings, such anatomic evidence may precipitate an ill-advised cascade of clinical interventions, especially when the tests are done too early in the clinical course or in the absence of surgical indications. As the authors of an article on CT warned, "the mere finding of abnormal CT results in the absence of appropriate clinical findings can lead to so-called exploratory back surgery, with all its disastrous con-

TABLE 8. *Representative estimates of test accuracy for the diagnosis of herniated discs*

Test, source	Sensitivity	Specifity	Positive predictive value, high prior probability[a]	Negative predictive value, high prior probability[a]	Positive predictive value, low prior probability[b]	Negative predictive value, low prior probability[b]
Ipsilateral SLR, 9	0.80	0.40	0.67	0.57	0.04	0.99
Crossed SLR, 9	0.25	0.90	0.79	0.44	0.07	0.98
Impaired ankle reflex, 9	0.50	0.60	0.65	0.44	0.04	0.98
Plain CT, 31, 35	0.90	0.70	0.82	0.82	0.08	0.996
MRI, 3,31	0.90	0.70	0.82	0.82	0.08	0.996
CT myelography, 31	0.90	0.70	0.82	0.82	0.08	0.996
Thermography, 15	0.90	0.60	0.77	0.80	0.07	0.995

[a] High prior probablity = 60% likelihood of herniated disc before test; typical of a patient with sciatica, positive straight leg raising, and poor response to conservative therapy.
[b] Low prior probability=3%; typical of a patient with no sciatica or neurologic signs/symptoms.
SLR, straight leg raising; CT, computed tomography; MRI, magnetic resonance imaging.

sequences." These results also suggest that physicians who seek to reassure themselves, reassure their patients, or practice defensive medicine may be exposing their patients and themselves to greater risk by doing these tests than by avoiding unnecessary imaging.

Table 8 also demonstrates that plain CT, MRI, and CT myelography have roughly equivalent sensitivities and specificities. Thornbury et al. even employed ROC curves to compare these tests and could identify little difference. Thus, the choice at this time may often depend on factors other than test accuracy, including accessibility, cost, and invasiveness. Thornbury and his colleagues suggested that, where the probability of a herniated disc is moderate, a plain CT examination is most appropriate, based largely on cost. In situations where herniated disc is more likely and where CT myelography would have once been the test of choice, they now recommend using MRI (based largely on its noninvasiveness and its sensitivity for rare neural tumors).

Table 9 provides estimates of the accuracy of several tests for spinal stenosis.

Again, plain CT and MRI appear to have roughly equivalent levels of accuracy. In this case, both tests appear to be superior to plain myelography, but there have been few studies of CT myelography. In the few cases where results from CT myelography have been compared with plain CT and MRI, sensitivity seemed comparable.

Data on the accuracy of tests for spinal malignancies and infections are even more sparse. Table 10 shows some data on the accuracy of history and physical examination and plain x-ray. It can be seen that plain x-ray films are highly specific, though relatively insensitive. Li and Poon studied the accuracy of MRI for detecting cancer as a cause of spinal cord and cauda equina compression. They reported a sensitivity of 93% and specificity of 97%. In addition, they reported that MRI was highly successful in distinguishing between benign and malignant compression fractures, using a signal intensity ratio. For this purpose, they reported a sensitivity of almost 98% and a specificity of 100%.

Another study used specific imaging sequences to study the presence of small

TABLE 9. *Representative estimates of test accuracy for the diagnosis of spinal stenosis*

Test, source	Sensitivity	Specifity	Positive predictive value, high prior probability[a]	Negative predictive value, high prior probability[a]	Positive predictive value, low prior probability[b]	Negative predictive value, low prior probability[b]
Plain CT, 16	0.90	0.80–0.95	0.87	0.84	0.12	0.996
MRI, 16	0.90	0.75–0.95	0.87	0.84	0.12	0.996
Myelography, 16	0.77	0.70	0.79	0.67	0.07	0.990

[a] High prior probablity = 60% likelihood of spinal stenosis before test; typical of a patient over age 50 with pseudoclaudication.

[b] Low prior probability = 3%; typical of a patient with no sciatica or neurologic signs/symptoms.

TABLE 10. *Representative estimates of test accuracy for the diagnosis of metastatic cancer (8)*

Test, references	Sensitivity	Specifity	Positive predictive value, prior probability = 0.20	Negative predictive value, prior probability = 0.20
Age . 50	0.77	0.71	0.10	0.93
Previous cancer	0.31	0.98	0.79	0.85
No relief, bed rest	> 0.90	0.46	0.29	0.95
ESR . 50 mm/h	0.56	0.97	0.82	0.90
Plain x-ray: lytic or blastic lesions	0.60	0.995	0.97	0.91
Plain x-ray: compression fracture or lytic/blastic lesion	0.70	0.95	0.78	0.93

ESR, erythrocyte sedimentation rate.

metastases among patients with a known primary tumor and progressive back pain who were suspected of having spinal metastases. Out of 40 patients, 21 showed metastases by MRI, and all 21 had biopsy confirmation of the diagnosis. Thus, the predictive value of a positive test was high (in this case 100%), although we cannot quantify the sensitivity and specificity since biopsies were not obtained on every patient. However, plain x-ray films and CT scans were normal in all 40 patients, so that MRI was substantially more sensitive.

In part because it is so rare, vertebral osteomyelitis is even less well studied with regard to test accuracy. However, in one recent study, MRI was found to have a sensitivity of 96% and specificity of 92%, while bone scanning had a sensitivity of 90% and specificity of 78%. Plain x-ray films had a sensitivity of 82%, but a specificity of only 57%. Thus, bone scanning and MRI were both superior to plain x-ray films, but MRI may be even more accurate than radionuclide bone scanning.

SUMMARY AND CONCLUSION

Diagnosis is inherently a probabilistic exercise. Before autopsy, we can rarely be absolutely certain about a diagnosis, and even autopsy cannot reveal whether a particular abnormality was actually a source of symptoms. The history, physical examination, and diagnostic tests are all aimed at raising or lowering the probability of various diagnoses as a cause of low back pain. Contrary to the misconception that imaging tests are infallible, we can see that all available diagnostic tests are imperfect. Thus, the correlation of clinical and imaging findings and the use of time and observation may be crucial in making optimal management decisions.

In many centers, it is commonplace to obtain multiple diagnostic tests on a patient, but we should question this practice. Aside from providing redundant information, multiple tests increase the probability of at least one positive result by chance alone and thus increase false-positive findings. Some critical observers believe that excessive diagnostic testing is one key factor leading to unnecessary treatments and iatrogenic problems.

The data presented here are only approximations of the accuracy of various diagnostic maneuvers, and they should be interpreted with some caution. The data on which they are based are often fragmentary, and many of the available studies have potential biases that may inflate the estimates of accuracy. Better studies of test accuracy are definitely needed, as is better evaluation of optimal sequences of diagnostic tests and indications for these tests.

ACKNOWLEDGMENTS

Supported in part by Grant HS-06344 from the Agency for Health Care Policy and Research (the Back Pain Outcome Assessment Team) and the Northwest Health Services Research and Development Field Program, Seattle VA Medical Center.

SUGGESTED READING

1. Aronson HA, Dunsmore RH. Herniated upper lumbar discs. *J Bone Joint Surg [Am]* 1963; 45:311–317.
2. Avrahami E, Tadmor R, Dally O, Hadar H. Early MR demonstration of spinal metastases in patients with normal radiographs and CT and radionuclide bone scans. *J Comput Assist Tomogr* 1989;13:598–602.
3. Boden SD, Davis DO, Dina TS, Patronas NJ, Wiesel SW. Abnormal magnetic resonance scans of the lumbar spine in asymptomatic subjects: a prospective investigation. *J Bone Joint Surg [Am]* 1990;72A:403–408.
4. Carette S, Marcoux S, Truchon R, et al. A controlled trial of corticosteroid injections into facet joints for chronic low back pain. *New Engl J Med* 1991;325:1002–1007.
5. Centor RM. Signal detectability: the use of ROC curves and their analyses. *Med Decis Making* 1991;11:102–106.
6. Deyo RA. The reproducibility and accuracy of lumbar spine imaging studies. In: Wiesel S, ed. *The lumbar spine.* 2nd ed. Philadelphia: Saunders [*in press*].
7. Deyo RA, Haselkorn J, Hoffman R, Kent DL. Designing studies of diagnostic tests for low back pain or radiculopathy. *Spine,* 1994; 185:2057s–2065s.
8. Deyo RA, Diehl AK. Cancer as a cause of back pain: frequency, clinical presentation, and diagnostic strategies. *J Gen Intern Med* 1988;3:230–238.
9. Deyo RA, Rainville J, Kent DL. What can the history and physical examination tell us about low back pain? *JAMA* 1992;268:760–765.
10. Deyo RA, Tsui-Wu JY. Descriptive epidemiology of low-back pain and its related medical care in the United States. *Spine* 1987; 12:264–268.
11. Garvey TA, Marks MF, Wiesel SW. A prospective randomized double-blind evaluation of trigger point injection therapy for low back pain. *Spine* 1989;14:962–964.
12. Gran JT. An epidemiological survey of the signs and symptoms of ankylosing spondylitis. *Clin Rheumatol* 1985;4:161–164.
13. Hakelius A, Hindmarsh J. The significance of neurological signs and myelographic findings in the diagnosis of lumbar root compression. *Acta Orthop Scand* 1972;43:239–246.
14. Hart LG, Deyo RA. Physician office visits for low back pain: frequency, clinical evaluation, and treatment patterns from a U.S. national survey. *Spine,* in press.
15. Hoffman RM, Kent DL, Deyo RA. Diagnostic accuracy and clinical utility of thermography for lumbar radiculopathy: a meta-analysis. *Spine* 1991;16:623–628.
16. Kent DL, Haynor DR, Larson EB, Deyo RA. Diagnosis of lumbar spinal stenosis in adults: a meta-analysis of the accuracy of CT, MR, and myelography. *AJR* 1992;158:1135–1144.
17. Kortelainen P, Puranen J, Koivisto E, Lahde S. Symptoms and signs of sciatica and their relation to the localization of the lumbar disc herniation. *Spine* 1985;10:88–92.
18. Kosteljanetz M, Espersen JO, Halaburt H, Miletic T. Predictive value of clinical and surgical findings in patients with lumbargo-sciatica: a prospective study (part 1). *Acta Neurochir* 1972;48:234–238.

19. Li KC, Poon PY. Sensitivity and specificity of MRI in detecting malignant spinal cord compression and in distinguishing malignant from benign compression fractures of vertebrae. *Magnetic Resonance Imaging* 1988; 6:547–556.

20. Modic MT, Feiglin DH, Piraino DW, et al. Vertebral osteomyelitis: assessment using MR. *Radiology* 1985;157:157–166.

21. Morris EW, DiPaola M, Vallance R, Waddell G. Diagnosis and decision making in lumbar disk prolapse and nerve entrapment. *Spine* 1986;11:436–439.

22. Nachemson AL. The lumbar spine: an orthopaedic challenge. *Spine* 1976;1:59–71.

23. Nice DA, Riddle DL, Lamb L, Mayhew TP, Rucker K. Intertester reliability of judgement of the presence of trigger points in patients with low back pain. *Arch Phys Med Rehabil* 1992;73:893–898.

24. Oxman AD, Sackett DL, Guyatt GH, et al. Users' guides to the medical literature: I. How to get started. *JAMA* 1993;270:2093–2095.

25. Potter NA, Rothstein JM. Intertester reliability for selected clinical tests of the sacroiliac joint. *Phys Ther* 1985;65:1671–1675.

26. Quebec Task Force on Spinal Disorders: A scientific approach to the assessment and management of activity-related spinal disorders: a monograph for clinicians. *Spine* 1987; 12[Suppl 7]:S22–S30.

27. Russell AS, Maksymowych W, LeClercq S. Clinical examination of the sacroiliac joints: a prospective study. *Arthritis Rheum* 1981; 24:1575–1577.

28. Sackett DL. A primer on the precision and accuracy of the clinical examination. *JAMA* 1992;267:2638–2644.

29. Sackett DL, Haynes RB, Guyatt GH, Tugwell P. *Clinical epidemiology: a basic science for clinical medicine.* 2nd ed. Boston: Little Brown; 1991.

30. Spangfort EV. Lumbar disc herniation: a computer aided analysis of 2504 operations. *Acta Orthop Scand Suppl* 1972;142:1–93.

31. Thornbury JR, Fryback DG, Turski PA, et al. Disk-caused nerve compression in patients with acute low-back pain: diagnosis with MR, CT myelography, and plain CT. *Radiology* 1993;186:731–738.

32. Turner JA, Ersek M, Herron L, Deyo RA. Surgery for lumbar spine stenosis: attempted meta-analysis of the literature. *Spine* 1992; 17:1–8.

33. Waldvogel FA, Vasey H. Osteomyelitis: the past decade. *N Engl J Med* 1980;303:360–370.

34. White AA III, Gordon SL. Synopsis: workshop on idiopathic low back pain. *Spine* 1982;7:141–149.

35. Wiesel SW, Tsourmas N, et al. A study of computer assisted tomography: I. The incidence of positive CAT scans in an asymptomatic group of patients. *Spine* 1984;9: 549–551.

5

History and Physical Examination

Jeffrey D. Klein and *Steven R. Garfin

*Department of Orthopaedic Surgery, Hospital for Joint Diseases Orthopaedic Institute, New York, New York 10003, USA; and *Department of Orthopaedics, University of California at San Diego, San Diego, California 92103–8894, USA*

Key Points

- History and physical examination are essential.

- Lumbar spinal stenosis pain is relieved in the flexed, or seated position.

- Night pain is a "red flag" for tumor or infection.

- One must distinguish upper motor neuron from lower motor neuron findings.

- Sacral sparing indicates an incomplete spinal cord injury.

The history and physical examination of the spine includes a local examination of both the cervical and the thoracolumbar regions, as well as a thorough neurologic assessment. In each case the examination will be tempered by the specific clinical setting. There are special considerations, for example, in the case of trauma and spinal cord injury. In all instances, the physical examination must be preceded by a thorough history.

HISTORY

A careful history is essential in the evaluation of patients with spinal disorders. Most diagnoses are made, or at least suggested, at this stage. One must not only distinguish between the various primary disorders of the spine but also differentiate them from systemic processes affecting the spine, such as metastatic disease.

The location, quality, and chronicity of pain should be described. Coughing, sneezing, and straining cause an increase in intrathecal pressure. Radicular pain (pain along the sensory, or dermatomal, distribution of a spinal nerve root) that occurs during these activities suggests the possibility of nerve root compression by a space-occupying lesion of the spinal canal, such as a herniated disc. In the cervical spine, axially located neck pain must be distinguished from arm pain. A radicular pattern should be sought. In the lumbar spine, back pain must be distinguished from leg pain (sciatica). Classically, radiating sciatic type pain extends below the knee. However, S1 and, occasionally, L5 irritation can stop at the buttock or posterior thigh. The patient may describe radiation of pain from the back, over the hip, and down the thigh and leg to the foot. Exact localization should be sought. For example, pain radiating to the dorsum of the foot and the great toe suggests involvement of the L5 nerve root (Figs. 1 and 2).

Associated neurologic signs and symptoms should be sought. Dermatomal sensory loss, paresthesias, and localized motor weakness suggest compression of specific nerve roots. Any disturbance of bowel or bladder function is worrisome and demands immediate evaluation to exclude a diagnosis of a cauda equina syndrome. This is caused by compression of the nerve roots of the cauda equina by a space-occupying lesion, such as occurs with a large central disc herniation. The presentation includes bowel or bladder dysfunction, saddle anesthesia, and variable loss of motor and sensory function in the lower

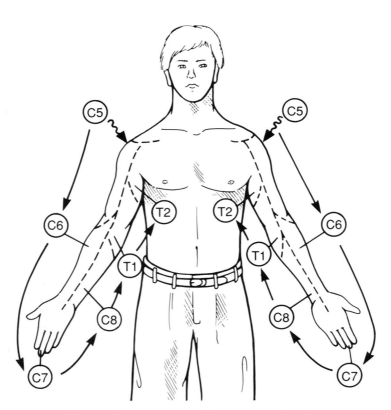

FIG. 1. Dermatomes of the upper extremity.

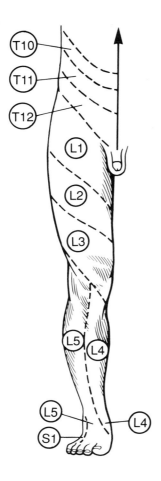

FIG. 2. Dermatomes of the lower extremity.

by the increased space available for the neural elements in the lumbar canal in this disorder when the spine is in flexion.

In the evaluation of low back pain, the type of work performed by the patient is important, as is any secondary gain associated with the condition. Age is also of importance when considering the diagnosis, as disc herniation is more common in adults younger than 55 and spinal stenosis is far more common in those older than 60 yr. In the trauma patient one should attempt to elicit the mechanism of injury, including the use of a seat belt in motor vehicle accidents.

Constant, unremitting pain is suggestive of tumor or infection. Night pain is also classically associated with these medically significant diseases. Concurrent symptoms such as fever, malaise, and weight loss suggest a systemic process, such as tumor or infection.

Any previous or family history of spinal disorders should be noted. Concurrent medical and psychiatric illnesses are also important, as they may contribute to the symptoms and signs. Inflammatory arthritides commonly involve the axial skeleton and may lead to pain complaints, as well as focal or generalized stiffness. Numerous visceral sources of back pain should be kept in mind as well. Peptic ulcers, cholecystitis, pancreatitis, retrocecal appendicitis, dissecting abdominal aortic aneurysms, pelvic inflammatory disease and endometriosis in the female patient, and prostate disorders in the male patient all can be sources of referred pain to the back. Angina, too, can be confused with cervical spine–related symptoms ("cervical angina").

extremities. Urgent evaluation by appropriate neurodiagnostic imaging followed by surgical intervention are indicated.

The pain of disc herniation tends to be worse when seated, presumably because of the increased intradiscal pressure in this position. In contrast, the neurogenic claudication of spinal stenosis is characterized by back and diffuse leg pain produced by walking and relieved by rest, including sitting down. This is explained

THE CERVICAL SPINE

Inspection

As in all areas of the physical examination, examination of the cervical spine begins with inspection. In this instance this includes observing the patient walk into the examination room. Gait, posture, and head position all offer clues as to underlying abnormalities.

The patient should be seated and the neck viewed from the front, sides, and back for deformities. Head tilt may signify a muscular torticollis secondary to traumatic or inflammatory involvement of the sternocleidomastoid muscle. In this case, the head tilts toward the ipsilateral shoulder and rotates toward the contralateral side. Head tilt may, however, reflect cerebellar dysfunction or an ophthalmologic disorder. In the younger patient one must consider congenital scoliosis or atlantoaxial rotatory subluxation. The latter is a rotational and/or translational deformity involving the 1st and 2nd cervical vertebrae, most often traumatic or inflammatory in nature.

It is extremely important, though frequently forgotten, to have the patient undress above the waist. This allows examination of the shoulder and back, anatomically related areas that can be sources of referred pain to the neck.

Palpation

The examination proceeds with anterior and posterior palpation of the bony and soft tissue structures of the neck. The hyoid bone lies anteriorly at the level of the C-3 vertebral body. The thyroid cartilage marks the level of the C-4 and C-5 vertebral bodies. The first cricoid ring lies anterior to the C-6 vertebral body. The thyroid gland lies over the thyroid cartilage at the C4-5 vertebral level in the anterior midline. Tenderness or swelling of the sternocleidomastoid muscle may be traumatic or inflammatory in origin and can result in torticollis.

Occasionally, a cervical rib may be palpable in the supraclavicular fossa. This anomaly can be associated with thoracic outlet syndrome, an entity characterized by intermittent vascular or neurologic compromise of the upper extremity due to compression of the subclavian vessels or the lower two nerve roots (C8, T1) of the brachial plexus. Additionally, compression of these neurovascular structures as they pass between the scalenus anticus and scalenus medius muscles can also cause this syndrome. One maneuver to assess this compression is *Adson's test.* For this, the patient's radial pulse is palpated and noted before and after the arm is passively abducted, extended, and externally rotated. The patient is then told to turn his or her head toward the arm in question. Diminution or loss of the pulse suggests compression of the subclavian artery and a possible diagnosis of thoracic outlet syndrome.

Posteriorly, the spinous processes and interspinous ligaments should be assessed for tenderness. Such tenderness in the trauma patient suggests posterior ligamentous injury or a spinous process fracture. Generalized posterior cervical tenderness may also signify simple muscular strain. The spinous processes are aligned in the midline in the normal subject. A shift in alignment may signify a unilateral facet dislocation or a spinous process fracture. However, these changes in alignment, or even the absolute levels of the structures, are often not easily discernible without radiographs. The C-7 and T-1 spinous processes are usually the most prominent and may serve as useful bony landmarks to the respective vertebral levels posteriorly.

One may also encounter tenderness posterolaterally over the trapezius muscle. This may be due to direct injury or spasm secondary to trauma or may be referred from an underlying cervical condition such as spondylosis, tumor, or infection. The greater occipital nerves represent the dorsal rami of C-2 and may be tender at the base of the skull.

Range of Motion

Active and passive range of motion should be noted. Qualitative descriptions of motion are probably more reproducible than specific numeric measurements. Measurement of the distance of the chin to the sternum in flexion and of the occiput to the dorsal spine in extension are helpful. This can be described in terms of fingerbreadths or measured with a ruler. The normal patient, for example, can touch chin to chest in flexion and bring the occiput to within three or four fingerbreadths of the dorsal spine in extension. Alternatively, a goniometer or inclinometer can be used for more precise angular measurements. Normal rotation is almost 90° (the chin should align with the shoulder), and lateral bending approaches 45°. Approximately 50% of the flexion and extension in the cervical spine occurs at the occiput-C1 articulation, and 50% of the rotation occurs across the C1-2 motion segment.

Provocative Testing

The *cervical compression test* is a provocative maneuver performed by applying axial pressure on the top of the patient's head. *Spurling's test* includes compression of the head with the neck extended and rotated to the site of the radicular pain. Positive responses to these tests include neck and, more importantly, arm pain (note a radicular pattern if present). This is generally seen in the setting of disc herniation or neuroforaminal encroachment of the nerve root. The *cervical distraction test* is performed by gradually distracting the patient's head. Patients with nerve root compression from herniated discs or neuroforaminal narrowing may note diminution of pain, as the distraction maneuver tends to enlarge the neuroforamen and decrease the load across the facet joints.

Upper Extremity Evaluation

Directly related to the physical examination of the cervical spine is the examination of the upper extremity by neurologic levels. Table 1 summarizes the

TABLE 1. *Muscle grading*

Muscle gradations	Description
5—Normal	Motion against gravity with full resistance
4—Good	Motion against gravity with some resistance
3—Fair	Motion against gravity
2—Poor	Motion with gravity eliminated
1—Trace	Evidence of slight contractility; no joint motion
0—Zero	No evidence of contractility

standard system for grading muscle strength. Motor, sensory, and reflex activity, if appropriate, should be assessed at each root level. The critical importance of this examination warrants a review of these levels at this stage.

The C5 nerve root innervates the deltoid muscle (shoulder abduction) and, along with C6, the biceps muscle (elbow flexion). It supplies sensation to the lateral arm (over the shoulder) and is primarily responsible for the biceps reflex (Fig. 3). The C6 root innervates the wrist extensors and, along with C5, the biceps muscle. The C6 sensory distribution includes the lateral forearm, the thumb, the index finger, and occasionally part of the middle finger. The posterior ramus

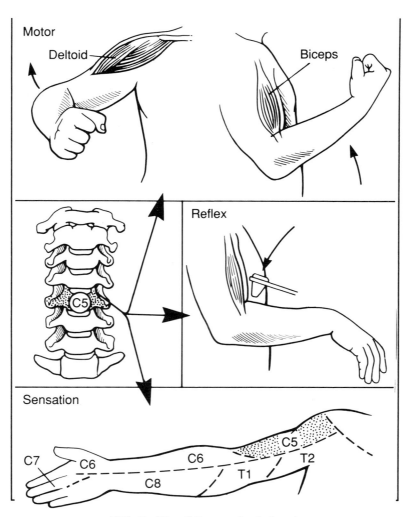

FIG. 3. The C5 neurologic level.

of C6, as well as those of C7 and C8, supply sensation to the region overlying the scapula. The associated reflex at this level is the brachioradialis (Fig. 4). The C7 motor distribution includes the triceps muscle (elbow extension), the wrist flexors, and the finger extensors. C7 provides sensation to the middle finger and is primarily responsible for the triceps reflex (Fig. 5). The C8 neurologic level includes motor innervation of the long finger flexors and the interossei. The sensory supply is to the ulnar side of the hand and the distal half of the ulnar aspect of the forearm. There is no reflex test for the C8 level (Fig. 6). The T1 level includes motor innervation of the interossei. Sensory supply is to the ulnar side of the

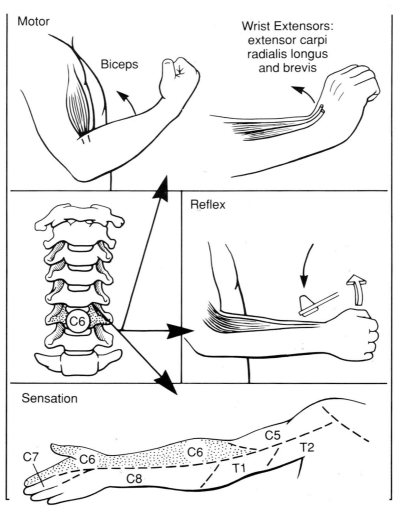

FIG. 4. The C6 neurologic level.

proximal forearm and distal arm. There is no associated deep tendon reflex (Fig. 7). Figure 1 demonstrates the sensory supply of the upper extremity by root level. Table 2 summarizes the neurologic levels of the upper extremity. It is important to note that the C4 sensory distribution includes the upper anterior chest wall. This is often confusing since thoracic innervation occurs immediately below. The remainder of the cervical roots (C5, C6, C7, C8) and the T1 root are, as noted above, represented along the arm and into the axilla. This distribution is related to the growth of the limb buds during embryonic development.

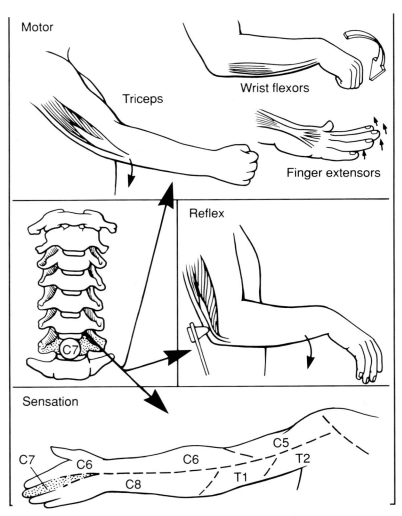

FIG. 5. The C7 neurologic level.

Anatomy

The nerve roots in the cervical spine exit above the pedicle of the correspondingly numbered vertebrae. There are eight cervical nerve roots and seven cervical vertebrae, thus changing this relationship at the cervicothoracic junction. Starting at T1 and throughout the remainder of the thoracolumbar spine, the numbered nerve root exits caudal to the pedicle of the corresponding vertebra. This has clinical implications in the evaluation of herniated discs. A typical posterolateral cervical disc herniation impinges on the nerve root exiting at the

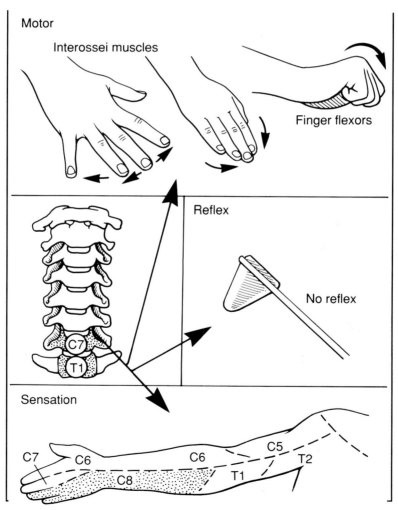

FIG. 6. The C8 neurologic level.

level of the disc. For example, a disc herniation at the C4-5 level compresses the C5 nerve root, and a C7-T1 herniated disc compromises the C8 root (Fig. 8). Occasionally, one may encounter an inconsistent or confusing level of neurologic involvement. In such a case, consider the possibility of a prefixed (begins at C4) or postfixed (begins at C6) brachial plexus.

Pathologic Reflexes

If the clinical setting warrants (trauma, rheumatoid arthritis, cervical spondylosis), it is important to test for pathologic

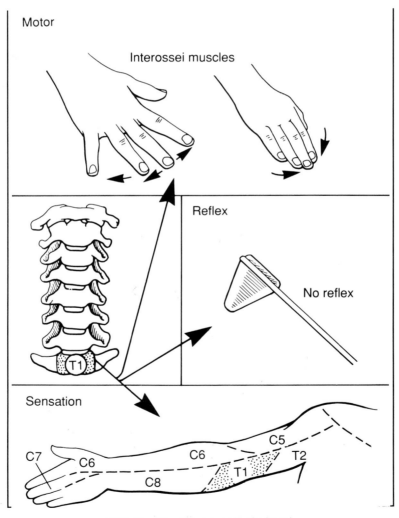

FIG. 7. The T1 neurologic level.

TABLE 2. *Neurologic levels of the upper extremity*

Root	Reflex	Muscles	Sensation
C5	Biceps reflex	Deltoid Biceps	Lateral arm (Axillary nerve)
C6	Brachioradialis Reflex	Wrist extension Biceps	Lateral forearm Musculocutaneous nerve)
C7	Triceps reflex Finger extension	Wrist flexors Triceps	Middle finger
C8	— Hand intrinsics	Finger flexion (Medial antebrachial cutaneous nerve)	Medial forearm
T1	—	Hand intrinsics	Medial arm (medial brachial cutaneous nerve)

upper motor neuron reflexes in both the upper and lower extremities, as well as other signs of myelopathy or spinal cord damage. *L'hermitte's sign* is characterized by shock-like pains radiating down the arms or legs with flexion of the neck.

Babinski's test involves firmly stroking the plantar surface of the foot with a sharp instrument, starting from the heel and proceeding distally along the lateral aspect of the sole and then medially across the forefoot. The normal, or neg-

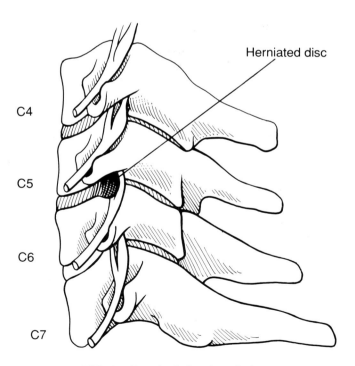

FIG. 8. Cervical disc herniation.

ative, response consists of no movement or downward motion of the toes. A positive response consists of extension of the great toe and spreading (fanning) of the lesser toes. *Oppenheim's sign* is tested for by firmly running one's finger distally along the crest of the tibia, with a positive response being the same as for the Babinski test. This test is sometimes better tolerated than Babinski's test by those patients with very sensitive feet.

Generalized hyperreflexia is also associated with myelopathy (spinal cord compression), especially when in conjunction with a positive Babinski sign. *Clonus* is a rhythmic, repetitive oscillation of the foot at the ankle in response to sudden, maintained dorsiflexion of the foot and stretching of the tendo achillis. The presence of clonus, too, is suggestive of myelopathy. *Hoffman's sign* is a pathologic reflex that is elicited in the upper extremity and is seen in association with patients having cervical myelopathy. The hand is held in a com-

fortable resting position and the nail of the middle finger is "flicked." A positive reaction consists of flexion of the terminal phalanx of the thumb and index finger (Fig. 9). If one elicits pathologic reflexes in the lower extremity and Hoffman's sign is negative, this may suggest that the problem lies below the level of the cervical spinal cord. This would be further supported by hyperreflexia limited to the lower extremities.

THE THORACIC AND LUMBAR SPINE

Physical examination of the thoracic and lumbar spine includes observation of the gait and general movements of the patient. Any splinting, antalgia, circumduction, "drop foot gait," Trendelenburg gait, or awkward motions should be noted. Further inspection with the patient disrobed should note any skin markings or hairy patches at the base of the spine. These may signify a benign spina bifida

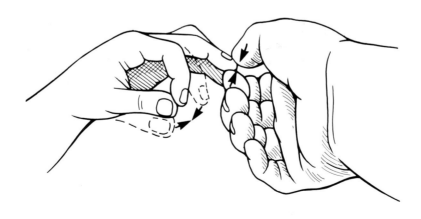

FIG. 9. Hoffman's sign.

or be related to a more significant anomaly, such as a diastematomyelia or a tethered spinal cord in the child.

The overall posture should be assessed and any deformities in the sagittal or coronal plane described. Scoliosis may be idiopathic or congenital in the child. Idiopathic scoliosis in the child is generally painless. Complaints of pain should prompt one to consider other concurrent diagnoses. An acute onset of scoliosis in an adult suggests either sciatica or tumor. In the child, serial clinical and radiographic examinations are needed to document evidence of progression of any deformity. In the *forward bend test,* the examiner kneels in front and then behind the patient while the patient flexes forward at the waist, drops their hands, and flexes their neck. One inspects the spinal alignment and notes any rib asymmetry, which reflects the rotational deformity seen concurrently with scoliosis. By sighting down the spine, one can roughly measure the height of the rib prominence. A more accurate and reproducible assessment of the rotational deformity can be made with a scoliometer or inclinometer.

The overall balance of the spine can be assessed by dropping a plumb line (a weighted string or tape measure) from the C-7 vertebra or the occipital prominence. This straight line normally aligns with the gluteal cleft, indicating that the trunk is centered over the pelvis ("in balance"). Distance in centimeters, lateral to the cleft, should be recorded. Another method to assess alignment is simply to note the position of the trunk relative to the pelvis. It is important to exclude leg length inequality as a cause of pelvic

obliquity and scoliosis. True leg lengths are generally measured from the ipsilateral anterior superior iliac spine to the medial malleolus, with the patient supine. The apparent or functional leg length is measured from the umbilicus to the medial malleolus. Apparent leg length inequality may be secondary to fixed pelvic obliquity or due to an adduction or flexion deformity of the hip.

The iliac crest and the posterior superior iliac spine are posterior bony landmarks that can aid in establishing approximate vertebral levels. The top of the iliac crest usually lies at approximately the level of the L4-5 interspace, and the posterior superior iliac spine lies at the level of S-2. The spinous processes and interspinous ligaments (posterior midline) should be palpated and percussed for tenderness. Tenderness or a palpable gap in the trauma patient suggests ligamentous instability or fracture. A step-off across the spinous processes suggests the possibility of spondylolisthesis. The paraspinal muscles should be palpated, and any spasm or tenderness noted. Finally, the area over the sciatic nerve in the region of the sciatic notch should be palpated. Tenderness suggests irritation of contributing nerve roots, most commonly by a disc herniation but occasionally by muscle spasm or direct trauma to the nerve.

Anteriorly, in a thin patient, with deep pressure, one can palpate the sacral promontory and with difficulty the L-4, L-5, and S-1 vertebral bodies. Palpation of the anterior abdominal muscles with the patient in a partial sit-up position can detect weakness or asymmetry in these segmentally innervated muscles. One should take this opportunity to examine the abdomen (routine evaluation including tenderness, masses, organomegaly, and aortic enlargement) to exclude sources of referred pain to the back. A rectal examination is required in older patients to examine rectal sphincter tone, in the male patient to palpate the prostate gland, or in those complaining of coccygeal (tailbone) pain. A pelvic examination should be considered in the female patient to exclude other sources of referred low back pain.

Range of motion should be tested and here, as in the cervical spine, qualitative descriptions are useful. Flexion can be measured by having the patient bend as far forward as possible, with the knees held straight, and noting the distance from the floor to the fingertips. One can also estimate the motion in degrees or as a percentage of total normal motion. It is important to note that much of the apparent flexion in the lower back occurs through the hips. The modified *Schober's test* attempts to identify those patients with true limitation of motion in the lumbar spine. With the patient standing, a 15-cm span is measured over the lumbar spine, beginning 10 cm above and extending 5 cm below the L-5 spinous process. The test is considered positive if this span is not increased by at least 6 cm in full flexion. In *Burn's test* the patient is asked to kneel on a chair and retrieve an object held below his reach. Patients with low back pain are generally able to perform this task by flexing at the hip if necessary. Those who cannot perform this test may not be making a genuine effort to do so.

Flexion and extension in the thoracic spine is limited because of the small size of the discs, the restraint imposed by the rib cage, and the coronal orientation of the facets. Rotation, however, is greater than across the lumbar spine. In the lumbar spine, the larger discs, the absence of ribs, and the sagittal alignment of the facets allow a large flexion and extension arc, though rotation is limited. Lateral bending should also be tested and has particular relevance in scoliosis, where one is trying to distinguish between flexible and rigid curves.

Pain during or limitation of forward flexion is a rather nonspecific finding. Pain on extension or hyperextension also may be a nonspecific finding but can signify spondylolysis or spondylolisthesis in the younger, active patient. In an older individual, pain (particularly reproduction of leg pain complaints) on extension may be seen with spinal stenosis. Such patients often find relief in the flexed, or seated, position.

The examination of the thoracic and lumbar spine by neurologic levels should be routinely performed, as it is for the cervical spine. As noted above, thoracic motor function is assessed with the patient performing a partial sit-up, in order to detect any asymmetry in the segmentally innervated rectus abdominus muscles. The upper portions of these muscles are supplied by the T5-10 roots, and the lower portions are supplied by T10-L1. Weakness on one side only causes the umbilicus to move in the opposite direction (positive *Beevor's sign*). The sensory dermatomes of the trunk are depicted in Fig. 10. As a rough guide, the T4 dermatome lies at the level of the nipple line, T7 at the level of the xiphoid process, T10 at the umbilicus, and T12 at the inguinal crease. The superficial abdominal reflex is an upper motor neuron reflex based on the segmental innervation of the abdominal musculature. With the patient supine and relaxed, each quadrant of the abdomen is stroked. In the normal response, the umbilicus moves toward the stroked area. Lack of this superficial reflex suggests an upper motor neuron lesion. This is in contradistinction to the deep tendon reflexes, where increased reflexes would be expected in an upper motor neuron lesion.

Thoracic disc herniation is rare and when present tends to cause cord, as well as root, symptoms. If myelopathy is suspected from the clinical setting, pathologic

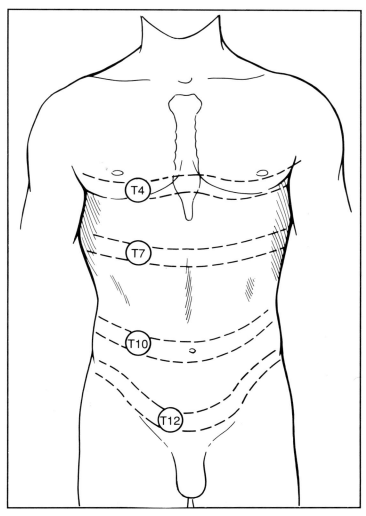

FIG. 10. Sensory dermatomes of the trunk.

upper motor neuron reflexes should be tested, as described for the cervical spine. In the adult patient with thoracic back and radicular pain, one should also consider herpes zoster (shingles), noting that pain may precede the vesicular eruption.

Lower Extremity Evaluation

The L1, L2, and L3 motor levels are tested by examining the iliopsoas mus-cle (hip flexion, primarily L1 and L2). The corresponding sensory distribution includes the anterior thigh below the inguinal ligament. The superficial cre-masteric reflex is another upper motor neuron reflex that tests the integrity of the T12 (efferent) and L1-2 (afferent) neurologic levels. An intact reflex is char-acterized by unilateral elevation of the scrotal sac when the skin of the ipsilat-eral inner thigh is stroked. The L2, L3,

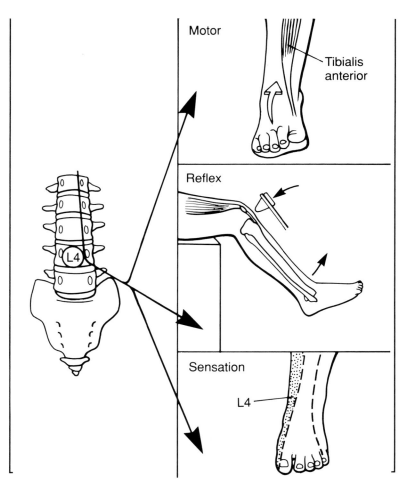

FIG. 11. The L4 neurologic level.

and L4 nerve roots innervate the quadriceps muscle (knee extension, primarily L3 and L4). The sensory distribution courses along the anterior and anterolateral thigh.

The L4 nerve root innervates the tibialis anterior muscle (foot dorsiflexion) in addition to the quadriceps. Heel walking is thus a test of the L4 motor level (additional contribution from the L5 innervated dorsiflexors of the great and lesser toes). The L4 root supplies sensation to the medial aspect of the leg and quite consistently to the skin overlying the medial malleolus. It is primarily responsible for the patellar reflex, though cross innervation occurs from L3 and, to a lesser extent, L2 (Fig. 11).

The L5 root innervates the extensor hallucis longus (great toe extension). The

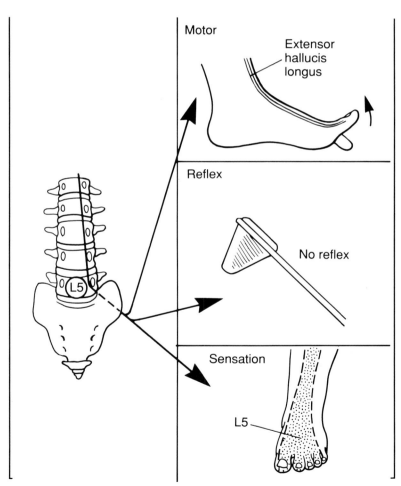

FIG. 12. The L5 neurologic level.

patient is seated with both feet on the floor and is asked to actively dorsiflex both great toes against resistance. Both toes are tested simultaneously to determine asymmetry of strength. The L5 root is also the primary innervation of the hip abductors (additional contribution from S1). In *Trendelenburg's test,* the patient is asked to stand on one leg and then the other, while the examiner sits behind the patient with his hands on the patient's iliac crests. Normally, the pelvis remains level during this maneuver. Any drop of the pelvis on the side opposite the stance leg constitutes a positive sign. A positive Trendelenburg sign implies weakness of the hip abductors on the weight-bearing side due to L5 root dysfunction or a primary pathologic condition of the hip joint. The patient should not be allowed to com-

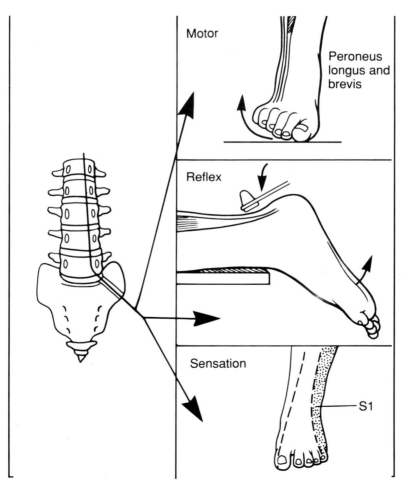

Motor

Peroneus longus and brevis

Reflex

Sensation

S1

FIG. 13. The S1 neurologic level.

pensate for abductor weakness by shifting the trunk over the stance leg during the test.

The L5 root provides sensation to the lateral aspect of the leg and the dorsum of the foot, including the great toe. The first web space is uniformly attributable to L5. The associated reflex at this level is the tibialis posterior, if present. It is, however, difficult to elicit, and this test is not routinely performed (Fig. 12).

The S1 level includes motor innervation to the peronei and, along with S2, the gastrocsoleus muscle. Toe walking, then, is an indication of the integrity of the S1 motor level. S1 provides sensation to the lateral aspect and sole of the foot, as well as the posterior leg. The associated reflex is that of the Achilles tendon (Fig. 13).

The S2, S3, and S4 levels supply the bladder as well as the intrinsic muscles of the foot. The foot should be examined for cavus (high arch) and claw toe deformities. The innervation of the bladder can be assessed with urodynamic evaluation, if necessary. These levels also supply perianal sensation and provide innervation for the superficial anal reflex. Figure 2 depicts the sensory dermatomes of the lower extremity. Table 3 summarizes the neurologic levels of the lower extremity.

The nerve roots of the lumbar spine exit below the pedicle of the correspondingly numbered vertebrae and above the discs, which are immediately caudal. A typical posterolateral disc herniation impinges on the nerve root that traverses over it, medial to the neuroforamen. For example, a disc herniation at the L4-5 level most often affects the L5 nerve root (Fig. 14). However, a disc herniation lateral to or at the neuroforamen can affect the exiting nerve root above (e.g., L4 for a far lateral L4-5 disc herniation), while a central herniation can affect one or more caudal nerve roots. A large central herniation is a common cause of the cauda equina syndrome and, unlike most other disc herniations, represents a surgical urgency.

Root tension signs are tests used to put the sciatic or femoral nerves on stretch. These are used primarily in the evaluation of the patient with suspected disc herniation and nerve root compression. The *straight-leg raising test* is performed with the patient supine or sitting on the examining table. The ankle is grasped and the leg lifted with the knee held in extension. A positive test reproduces the patient's radicular pain. The degree of hip flexion at which hip or leg pain is experienced should be noted.

TABLE 3. *Neurologic levels of the lower extremity*

Root	Reflex	Muscles	Sensation
L2	—	Iliopsoas	Anterior thigh, groin
L3	(Patellar reflex)	(Quadriceps)	Anterior and lateral thigh
L4	Patellar reflex	Anterior tibialis	Medial leg and medial foot; medial malleolus
L5	—	Extensor hallucis	Lateral leg and longus dorsum of foot; first web space
S1	Achilles reflex	Peroneus longus	Lateral foot; little toe and brevis

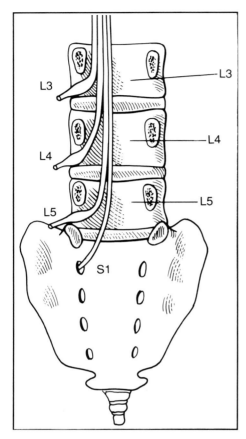

FIG. 14. Lumbar disc herniation.

uninvolved leg is elevated. A positive response reproduces pain in the opposite (involved) leg and suggests the possibility of an axillary disc herniation or a free fragment. The *femoral stretch test* is performed with the patient in either the prone or the lateral decubitus position and involves extension of the thigh at the hip with the knee flexed. Reproduction of the patient's pain (usually anterior or anterolateral thigh pain) is a tension sign suggesting involvement of the upper (L2, L3, and L4) nerve roots.

Sacroiliac joint abnormality can be a cause of low back pain. One test for this is the *Patrick* or *FABER* (flexion, abduction, external rotation) test. With the patient supine, the knee is flexed and the foot placed on the opposite patella. The flexed knee is then pushed by the examiner as far laterally as possible, and any increased pain in the region of the sacroiliac joint is noted (Fig. 15). The *pelvic rock test* is also performed supine and involves compression of the iliac crests toward the midline of the body. This, too, may elicit pain with derangement of the sacroiliac joint.

Hamstring pain and tightness may cause posterior thigh pain. If there is any question, the knee can be flexed slightly from maximum extension and the foot dorsiflexed (the *Lasegue maneuver*) to again put the sciatic nerve on stretch and reproduce the patient's pain. Alternatively, with the knee slightly flexed, pressure can be applied to the tibial nerve in the region of the popliteal fossa (the *bowstring test*). The *contralateral* (well leg) straight leg raising test is performed in the same fashion as the standard straight leg raising maneuver, except that the

The hip can also be a cause of referred pain to the back. This is further complicated by the fact that in older patients osteoarthritis of the hip frequently coexists with degenerative disease of the lumbar spine. Both can lead to hip and thigh pain. The former usually causes anterior groin and thigh pain proximal to the knee, while spinal stenosis is more often posterolateral, extending distal to the knee. Even with neurodiagnostic studies, however, these clinical situations can be confusing. Occasionally, injection of local anesthetic into the hip or, con-

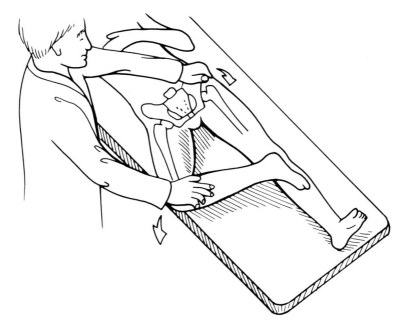

FIG. 15. The Patrick or FABER test.

versely, an epidural steroid injection can be helpful in sorting out the source of the pain.

When examining the patient with low back pain, it is important to check for any nonorganic physical signs such as described by Waddell et al. Five signs may identify those patients who have a significant psychologic or socioeconomic basis for their pain. *Nonorganic tenderness* may include either broad, superficial tenderness to light touch in the lumbar region and/or widespread deep tenderness in a nonanatomic distribution. *Simulation tests* suggest to the patient that a specific examination is being performed though, in fact, it is not. For example, low back pain produced with either axial loading of the skull or passive rotation of the shoulders and pelvis in the plane through the hips suggests involvement of nonorganic factors in the pain response. *Distraction tests* attempt to reproduce positive physical findings while the patient's attention is distracted. A positive supine straight-leg raising response may be suspect if the patient can flex his or her hip to 90° with the knee extended in the sitting position. This can be described to the patient as part of the routine "knee" examination. The supine straight leg raising test is more commonly performed, is described in all common texts, and can be learned by the patient.

Regional disturbances are sensory and motor abnormalities that involve multiple regions and are unexplained on a neuroanatomic basis. "Give way" weakness and sensory loss in a "stocking," rather

TABLE 4. *The Waddell signs*

Tenderness	(Superficial/nonanatomic)
Simulation	(Axial loading/rotation)
Distraction	(Straight leg raising)
Regional Overreaction	(Weakness/sensory)

SPECIAL CONSIDERATIONS IN TRAUMA AND SPINAL CORD INJURY

than dermatomal, distribution probably have a nonorganic component. *Overreaction* during examination is statistically the most important nonorganic physical sign. Disproportionate verbalization, inappropriate facial expression, tremor, collapsing, and sweating are all manifestations of this Waddell sign. The Waddell signs are summarized in Table 4.

In the case of spinal trauma, any subtle symptoms suggestive of neural injury, including transient numbness or paresthesias, must be sought out. Conversely, in a patient with known spinal cord injury, any evidence of transient motor or sensory function after the injury is important and suggests an incomplete cord injury. The trauma evaluation must include inspection of the entire spine. It is safest to use a backboard or a log-rolling maneuver during lateral turning.

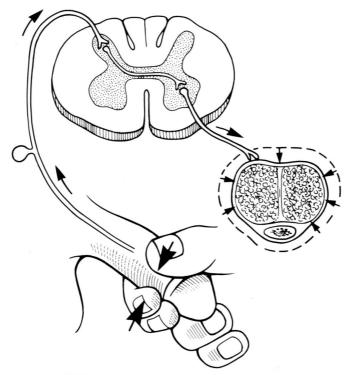

FIG. 16. The bulbocavernosus reflex.

Any tenderness, deformity, ecchymosis, or abrasions should be noted. Marks made by shoulder or seat belts should alert the examiner to the possibility of cervicothoracic or thoracolumbar spine injury, respectively. Suspect cervical spine trauma in any patient with significant craniofacial injury. One must be certain to evaluate the entire spine, even with a known injury, as the incidence of noncontiguous spinal fractures is estimated at 5% to 10%. A careful neurologic examination is obviously critical in the setting of spinal cord injury. The exam should be repeated serially to note any improvement or deterioration in the neurologic status.

After spinal cord injury, a patient enters a period of variable length termed *spinal shock,* which is characterized by spinal cord dysfunction based on physiologic, rather than structural, disruption. The resolution of spinal shock is marked by the return of the reflex arcs below the level of injury. This is most commonly tested by the bulbocavernosus reflex, which returns in 24 to 48 hours in 90% of patients. This reflex is mediated by the S3 and S4 nerve roots and involves squeezing, or pulling, the glans penis in the male or the clitoris in the female and noting contraction of the anal sphincter. This is sometimes easily performed by simply pulling on a Foley catheter (Fig. 16).

It is critical to distinguish between complete and incomplete neurologic deficit as early as possible. Any evidence of motor function or sensory sparing below the level of spinal cord injury denotes an incomplete deficit and offers the hope of some functional recovery. This determination cannot be made until the period of spinal shock has ended (return of the bulbocavernosus reflex or an elapsed time of more than 48 hr). Functional motor recovery is seen only rarely in patients presenting with complete neurologic deficits.

Often the only indication that a spinal cord injury is incomplete is preservation of sacral function. Sacral sparing indicates at least some structural continuity of the long tracts and, thus, a chance for functional recovery. Findings may include perianal sensation, some rectal tone, and great toe flexion. Figure 17 depicts the cross-sectional anatomy of the cervical spinal cord. The sacral structures are the most peripherally placed in both the lateral corticospinal tracts and the posterior columns. This provides the anatomic basis for sacral sparing, as the peripheral sacral elements are commonly preserved despite damage to the central fibers of the spinal cord. Documentation of the presence or absence of sacral sparing is important prognostically in the evaluation of the patient with spinal cord injury.

The various specific types of "incomplete" neurologic syndromes are described in Table 5. The central cord syndrome is common (particularly in older patients) and is characterized by sacral sparing and greater involvement of the upper extremity than the lower extremity. Some functional recovery can be expected in approximately 75% of these patients. The anterior cord syndrome is relatively uncommon and is characterized by a complete motor deficit below the level of injury and a very poor prognosis for functional recovery. In this instance, posterior column function (deep pressure, vibration, and proprioception) are usu-

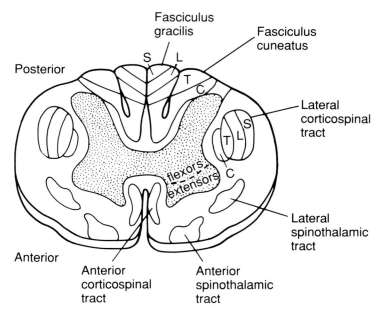

FIG. 17. Cross-section of the spinal cord in the cervical region.

ally intact. The Brown-Sequard syndrome is characterized by ipsilateral motor deficit and contralateral pain and temperature loss, usually two levels below the insult. This is uncommon, is usually secondary to penetrating trauma to the cord through a lateral "approach," and

carries the best prognosis, with greater than 90% functional recovery.

Imaging and Other Diagnostic Testing

The evaluation of the patient with spinal cord trauma proceeds with radi-

TABLE 5. *Incomplete cord syndromes*

Syndrome	Frequency	Description	Functional recovery
Central	Most common	Usually quadriplegic with sacral sparing. Upper extremities affected more than lower	75%
Anterior	Common	Complete motor deficit. Trunk and lower extremity deep pressure and proprioception preserved	10%
Posterior	Rare	Loss of deep pressure, deep pain, and proprioception	
Brown-Sequard	Uncommon	Ipsilateral motor deficit. Contralateral pain and temperature deficit	>90%

ographic and, ultimately, neurodiagnostic studies. Nonetheless, the focus of the initial assessment of these patients remains an accurate history and thorough physical examination. These are essential to minimize the risk of further neurologic injury and maximize the potential for neurologic recovery.

SUGGESTED READING

1. Bohlman HH. Acute fractures and dislocations of the cervical spine: an analysis of three hundred hospitalized patients and review of the literature. *J Bone Joint Surg [Am]* 1979; 61A:1119–1142.
2. Bracken MB, Shepard MJ, Hellenbrand KG, et al. Methylprednisolone and neurological function 1 year after spinal cord injury: results of the National Acute Spinal Cord Injury Study. *J Neurosurg* 1985;63:704–713.
3. Evanski PM, Carver D, Nehemkis A, Waugh TR. The Burns' test in low back pain. *CORR* 1979;140: 42–44.
4. Keenen TL, Benson DR. Initial evaluation of the spine-injured patient. In: Browner BD, Jupiter JB, Levine AM, Trafton PG, eds. *Skeletal trauma.* Philadelphia: WB Saunders; 1992:585–604.
5. Kewalramani LS, Taylor RG. Multiple noncontiguous injuries to the spine. *Acta Orthop Scand* 1976;47:52–58.
6. MaCrae IF, Wright V. Measurement of back movement. *Ann Rheum Dis* 1969;28:584–589.
7. McGuire RA, Neville S, Green BA, et al. Spinal instability and the log-rolling maneuver. *J Trauma* 1987;27:525– 531.
8. Moore KL. *The developing human: clinically oriented embryology.* Philadelphia: WB Saunders; 1977.
9. Scham SM, Taylor TKF. Tension signs in lumbar disc prolapse. *CORR* 1971;75:195–204.
10. Spratt KF, Lehmann TR, Weinstein JN, Colby H. A new approach to the low back physical examination: behavioral assessment of mechanical signs. *Spine* 1990;15(2):96–102.
11. Stauffer ES. Diagnosis and prognosis of acute cervical spinal cord injury. *CORR* 1975; 112:9–15.
12. Waddell G, McCulloch JA, Kummel E, et al. Non-organic physical signs in low-back pain. *Spine* 1980;5:117–125.

6

Diagnostic Imaging of the Spine

Scott D. Boden

*Department of Orthopaedic Surgery, Emory University School of Medicine,
The Emory Spine Center, Decatur, Georgia 30033, USA*

Key Points ━━━━━━━━━━━━━━━━━━━━━━━━━━━━━━━

- The most common misconception regarding spinal imaging is that these sophisticated tests are foolproof in detecting disease and guiding treatment.

- Imaging abnormalities must be correlated with historical and physical findings.

- Radiographs must be interpreted with an awareness of the wide variations among normal people and the frequent findings of degenerative changes in asymptomatic people.

- Thirty-four percent of asymptomatic people have abnormal CT scans; 20% to 25% of asymptomatic people have abnormal MRI scans.

- When to order a test is as important as what test to order.

- Errors in decision making are generally not related to misinterpretation of imaging studies but failure to integrate them with clinical information.

The most common and dangerous misconception about spinal imaging is that the increasingly sophisticated tests that are now available are foolproof in detecting spinal disease and guiding treatment. Actually, nothing could be farther from the truth. Despite the increased sophistication and detail that we have with modern imaging techniques, there is still a high frequency of false-positive findings. Therefore, there is no substitute for a detailed history and physical examination, and it is essential that any imaging abnormalities be correlated with the historical and physical findings.

Diagnostic tests should be used to confirm the core of information gathered from a thorough history and physical examination. Several imaging techniques are available, including plain film radiography, discography, myelography, computed tomography, and magnetic resonance imaging. While each of these tests has a place in the algorithm of the evaluation of neck and back problems, none should be used for general screening, since most are overly sensitive and relatively nonspecific. Many of the iatrogenic catastrophes in the management of acute neck and low back pain can be attributed directly to excessive reliance on diagnostic studies without positive clinical correlation.

THE STRENGTHS AND WEAKNESSES OF IMAGING TECHNIQUES

To evaluate the true clinical value of any diagnostic study, one must know its sensitivity (false negatives) and specificity (false positives). The specificity, or false-positive rate, is usually measured in a population of symptomatic patients who have undergone surgery. However, often there is a much higher rate of false positives when an asymptomatic group is studied. Stated more simply, the sensitivity is the ability of a test to detect disease when it is present. The specificity is the ability of a test to remain negative in the absence of clinical disease. The accuracy of any single test increases when it is combined with a second or third diagnostic study. The physician's challenge is to select diagnostic tests on the basis of

their performance characteristics so that the correct diagnosis is obtained with the least cost and morbidity.

Plain Radiographs

Degenerative changes develop in the cervical spine and surrounding tissues as part of the aging process. In the elderly the radiographic manifestations of cervical spondylosis occur with such regularity that they may not be related to symptoms. In many instances it is difficult to verify the clinical symptoms or the sequelae of the degenerative changes of cervical spondylosis. There is often no direct relationship between symptoms and the radiographic changes of degenerative disc disease in the cervical spine.

Although radiographic evidence of chronic disc degeneration is common in middle age, it is almost universal in the elderly. Degenerative disc disease in the cervical spine is usually not seen as an isolated finding, but rather as part of a process that affects the structure of the entire cervical spine (Fig. 1). The most commonly affected level is C5-6, with 86% of cadaveric specimens having observable abnormalities. C6-7 was the level next most frequently affected by chronic disc degeneration. By age 65, 95% of men and 70% of women have at least one degenerative change on their plain radiographs of the cervical spine. Anterior osteophyte formation (spurs) and disc space narrowing are the most common findings.

Radiographs must be interpreted with an awareness of the wide variations among normal patients as well as the frequent findings of degenerative changes

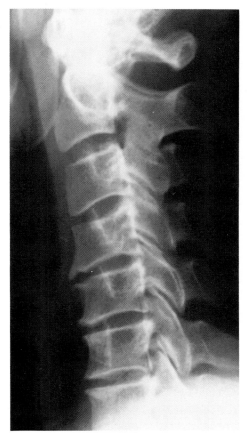

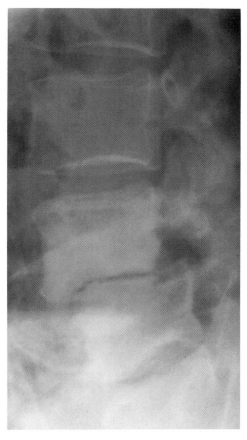

FIG. 1. Lateral cervical radiograph demonstrates loss of normal lordosis as well as degeneration of the C4-5, C5-6, and C6-7 disc spaces evidenced by loss of the normal progressive increase in disc height from cephalad to caudad and the spurs seen at C4-5.

FIG. 2. Lateral lumbar radiograph demonstrates a forward slip of L-4 on L-5 due to a degenerative spondylolisthesis at that level. There is loss of disc space height and resulting foraminal stenosis compared with the uninvolved levels.

in asymptomatic patients. Friedenberg and Miller (4) found that 35% of entirely asymptomatic patients had radiographic evidence of cervical spondylosis.

A similar scenario occurs with plain radiographs of the lumbar spine (Fig. 2).

Degenerative changes such as disc space narrowing, traction osteophytes, endplate sclerosis, and the vacuum disc phenomenon (a lucency in the disc space) are quite prevalent in middle aged and older individuals. Unfortunately, these radiographic findings do not correlate well with clinical symptoms. In fact, low back radiographs have been removed from most pre-employment screening physical examinations because of their inability to predict patients with low back problems. Plain radiographs are useful for the detection of signs of infection, bone tumors, and malalignment as a result of instability. Instability in the cervical spine is extremely rare, except after trauma and in patients with rheumatoid arthritis with synovial pannus causing destruction of supporting ligaments. Occasionally, oblique radiographs of the cervical spine can be useful for detecting isolated foraminal stenosis (encroachment of bony spurs into the exit zone of the spinal nerve roots).

In the lumbar spine, in addition to detecting infection and tumor, plain radiographs are frequently utilized for the detection of instability. The precise definition of instability is somewhat controversial, but in general it may be considered to be more than 3.5 mm of horizontal translation on a lateral weight-bearing radiograph from extension to flexion. Angular instability may also be present if the disc space shows excessive collapse into kyphosis. The presence of instability in and of itself is not an indication for any type of aggressive management unless it can be clearly associated with the patient's symptoms.

The standard set of radiographs for the cervical spine should include the following views: anterior/posterior, lateral, open-mouth odontoid, and obliques. The standard plain radiograph series for the lumbar spine should include the following: anterior/posterior view, lateral view, and spot-lateral of the lumbosacral junction. Flexion/extension views are not necessary unless instability is suggested on the basis of history and physical findings. Similarly, oblique radiographs in the lumbar spine may be used to visualize the pars interarticularis but are also not routinely indicated unless a pars defect or fracture is suspected.

Discography

A discogram is an injection of dye into the intervertebral disc space that is usually performed under local anesthesia. An abnormal discogram occurs when the dye is not contained within the confines of the disc space and when the injection reproduces the character distribution of the patient's back or neck pain (Fig. 3). Discography has been used in the cervical spine since 1957 and in the lumbar spine since 1948 but remains a controversial diagnostic technique. Proponents of discography claim that it is sensitive and accurate in identifying patients who have neck or back pain due to intrinsic disc abnormality (so-called *internal disc derangement* or *discogenic pain*). Others question the validity of this diagnosis or, more accurately, question the ability of their being able to make the diagnosis reliably. Therefore, the significance of a positive test remains somewhat uncertain and the results of treatment based on this test somewhat unpredictable, leading to the continued controversy surrounding discography.

In 1968, a study in prison volunteers found that 37% of asymptomatic young men had positive discograms based on abnormal postdiscographic imaging (i.e., dye leaked outside the normal confines of the nucleus pulposus). More recently, a study performed at the University of Iowa showed that there were no positive discograms in a group of asymptomatic patients when pain reproduction was the criteria used to define a positive test. Currently, discography is best reserved as a secondary diagnostic study to be used when less invasive tests are negative or equivocal in the presence of persistent mechanical neck or low back pain that is refractory to aggressive nonoperative management.

Myelography

Myelography has long been the "gold standard" for measuring neural compression in both the cervical and the lumbar spine. Dye is injected into the dural sac and mixes with the cerebrospinal fluid. The outline of the contents of the dural sac can be visualized on radiographs. Any extradural mass, such as a herniated disc, shows up as a filling defect in the dye column, while an intrathecal mass may appear as an outwardly protruding defect (Fig. 4). Myelography is unable to differentiate disc

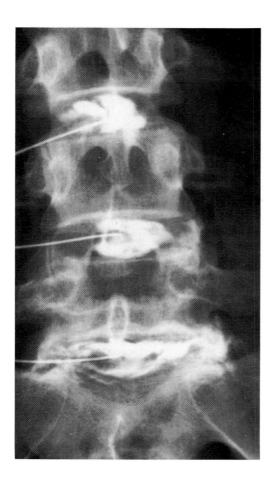

FIG. 3. Lumbar discogram demonstrates normal appearance at L3-4 and L4-5 but a torn annulus at L5-S1 with dye extravasation laterally.

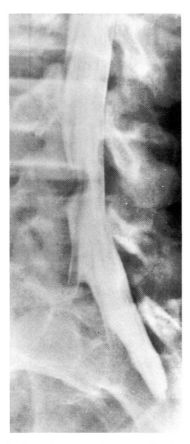

FIG. 4. Lumbar myelogram displays a filling defect at L4-5 from a herniated disc that displaces the exiting nerve root dorsally.

protrusion from bony, malignant, infectious, or other extradural encroachment on the spinal canal. The diagnostic accuracy of myelography is also questionable in cases of far lateral disease and in the lumbar spine at the L5-S1 level, where the epidural space may be large.

Originally, myelography was performed with oil-based dyes that caused a relatively high complication rate, including headache, nausea, vomiting, seizures, and arach-noiditis (intrathecal scarring of the nerve roots). More recently, water-soluble dye and nonionic contrast materials have allowed the detection of subtle changes in the contour or location of nerve roots without the increased risk of complications.

The primary advantage of myelography over other techniques, such as CT and MRI, is that myelography is a dynamic test that measures the ability of CSF to flow around any potential extradural lesions. In other words, a block on the myelogram implies a functional block in the ability of CSF to pass by the lesion and raises the level of severity of neural compression. It is difficult to ascertain this dynamic information on static examination, such as CT or MRI.

Although most studies report that the accuracy of CT and myelography is comparable, it has been shown in a blinded investigation that myelography may be more accurate (83% vs. 72%) in the diagnosis of herniated lumbar discs. In addition, myelography may have a lower false-positive rate and a higher false-negative rate than CT. Although expensive hospitalization was originally a deterrent to myelography, current procedures are tending more and more toward making this an outpatient procedure. The most common complication is spinal fluid leak, manifested by headache, nausea, vomiting, and occasionally dizziness; this can be managed with bed rest and occasionally requires a blood patch (placement of the patient's own blood epidurally at the site of the puncture to form a clot and control the CSF leak).

Myelography is not immune from the problem of false positives. In asymptomatic volunteers 21% have abnormal filling defects in their cervical myelograms and 24% have abnormal filling in their lumbar myelograms. Today myelography is rarely used as an individual investigation and is usually combined with post-myelographic computed tomography.

Computed Tomography

Computed tomography is currently the most versatile and widely available non-invasive technique for evaluating abnormalities of the spine. Multiple cross-sectional (axial) images of the spine are made at various levels and, with reformatting, coronal, sagittal, and three-dimensional images may be created. The CT scan

demonstrates not only the bony spine configuration, but also the soft tissue in graded shadings, so that ligaments, nerve roots, free fat, and intervertebral disc protrusions can be evaluated as they relate to their bony environment.

The CT scan is particularly useful for distinguishing between hard (osteophytes) and soft discs (herniated nucleus pulposus). In addition, CT is useful for localizing and finding the extent of neoplastic or infectious involvement in the spine, particularly as it relates to bony destruction and residual stability.

The clinical significance of CT/myelographic findings in cervical spondylosis was studied by Penning and associ-

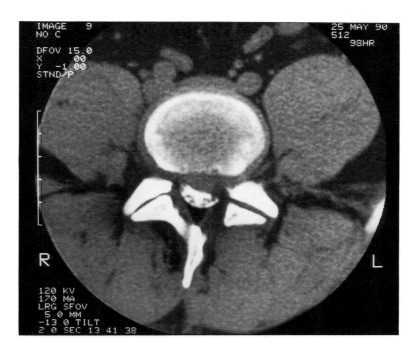

FIG. 5. Postmyelogram CT scan demonstrates a herniated disc at L4-5 (same patient as in Fig. 4) with compression of the dural sac and dorsal displacement of the left L5 nerve root.

ates. One hundred percent correlation was found between the side of disc herniation with occlusion of the intervertebral foramen and the side of nerve root symptoms. Symptoms of spinal cord compression were noted after the cross-sectional area of the spinal cord had been reduced by 30% or to a value of 60 mm^2 or less. Penning also observed that, in the presence of a normal conventional plain film myelogram, postmyelographic CT studies were rarely useful and in some cases may lead to false-positive interpretation of clinically irrelevant findings.

Several prospective comparisons of CT with myelography in the lumbar spine have demonstrated that CT is at least as sensitive (97% vs. 93%) and specific (80% vs. 76%) in the diagnosis of herniated lumbar discs. The sensitivity of CT appears to be enhanced by the addition of intradural contrast agent, which has been shown to demonstrate additional pathologic conditions in up to 30% of cases (Fig. 5). The routine axial CT scan is sometimes unable to demonstrate foraminal disc herniation, ventral facet hypertrophy, and endplate osteophytes. However, these findings can sometimes be seen with the use of multiplanar reformatting. The primary weakness of CT scanning remains its unreliability in demonstrating intrathecal abnormality (e.g., spinal cord tumors).

The CT scan is an extremely valuable diagnostic tool when it is used appropriately to confirm clinical findings. However, studies in asymptomatic volunteers have revealed the pitfalls of making clinical decisions on the basis of isolated CT scan findings. Despite many reports in the literature indicating that CT scans have

a mean accuracy of 90% in symptomatic patients, 34% of asymptomatic people have abnormal CT scans when reviewed by independent expert observers. The implication is that a patient with a negative history and physical examination for a spinal lesion has a 1 in 3 chance of having an abnormal CT scan of the lumbar spine. If a decision for surgery is based only on CT scan results, there is a 30% chance that the patient will undergo an unnecessary and unsuccessful operation. However, if the patient's clinical picture correlates well with the CT scan abnormalities, CT can be a useful confirmatory diagnostic tool and can increase the chances for a successful operation.

Magnetic Resonance Imaging

Magnetic resonance imaging is the newest diagnostic imaging technique for the spine. The image for different tissues is obtained by the detection of extremely small differences in proton density in a magnetic field bombarded with short pulses of radio waves that cause atoms to vibrate in a specific manner. Variations in proton density, radiofrequency, and relaxation time to the nonexcited state will modify the magnetic resonance (MR) image to highlight different tissues. Unlike CT and myelography, this approach does not require ionizing radiation or contrast agents. Multiplanar images are directly available.

A normal MR image of the spine will show the vertebral column, intervertebral discs, and spinal canal with the spinal cord in the sagittal view. On T2-weighted images (long relaxation and echo times), the intervertebral disc normally has high signal (white) but loses this signal with dehydration and early disc degeneration. The excellent anatomic resolution of MRI scans facilitates more precise description of disc disease. Disc herniations can be described as contained by the posterior longitudinal ligament, noncontained (extruded), or simply as a diffuse bulge (Fig. 6). In addition, the MRI scan has the ability to detect subtle tears in the annulus fibrosus that are undetectable by other imaging techniques. For the detection of routine degenerative disease, MRI is comparable to CT myelography. One area in which MRI is superior to all other techniques is the imaging of spinal tumors, both intradural and extradural, as well as the imaging of spinal infection. Gadolinium, an intravenous paramagnetic contrast agent, may enhance the dural/extradural interface and parenchymal lesions on T1-weighted images. Intramedullary abnormalities, such as syringomyelia, myelomalacia, intramedullary neoplasms, and demyelinating disease, are much better appreciated with MRI than with CT or myelography. In addition, the location and extent of infection is easily ascertained with MRI, largely because of the adjacent marrow edema, which is easily seen on T2-weighted MR images. In addition, epidural extension of either neoplasm or infection can be readily seen on axial images.

As with all other diagnostic imaging techniques, MRI has been shown to have a significant clinical false-positive rate in asymptomatic individuals. In the cervical spine, a variety of abnormalities were displayed in over 20% of asymptomatic subjects and a much higher percentage in subjects over the age of 40. Spinal cord impingement was seen in 10% to 15% of younger subjects and in 20% to 25% of older asymptomatic subjects. In the lumbar spine, 22% of asymptomatic subjects under age 60 and 57% of those over age 60 had a significant abnormality on their MR scan. In addition, the prevalence of disc degeneration on the T2-weighted MR images (so-called *dark disc disease*) was found to approach 98% in subjects over age 60. The importance of this observation is to emphasize that such findings are part of the normal spectrum of aging and should not be overinterpreted when seen on scans in symptomatic patients as they may not be the cause of any given patient's symptoms.

Bone Scan

Radionuclide imaging is a very good technique for the detection of bone abnormalities. Since bone is living tissue containing osteoblasts and osteoclasts, the activity of these cells is normally balanced; any process that disturbs the balance and results in increased bone production is associated with a greater concentration of radionuclide tracer on the bone scan. Interruption of blood flow to the bone will result in an absence (cold spot) of tracer on the scan (Fig. 7).

The most commonly used radiopharmaceutical for bone scanning is technetium-99m. Bone scan images are obtained with scintillation cameras that detect the production of gamma rays from different locations in the body. A large field-of-view camera can survey the entire skeleton, while close-up spot views are reserved for regions of clinical concern or suspicious areas seen on the total body image.

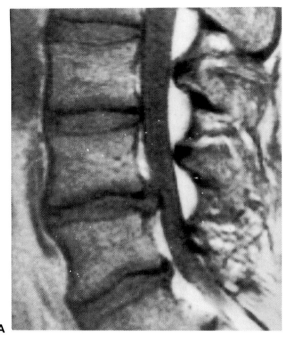

A

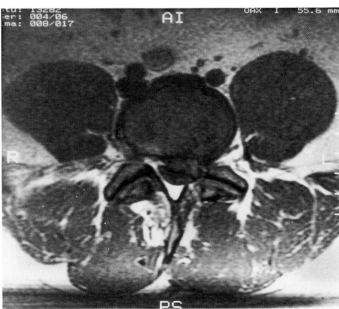

B

FIG. 6.A: Sagittal T1-weighted MR scan demonstrates a large herniated disc at L4-5 and a small contained disc herniation at L5-S1. **B:** Axial MR scan through L4-5 shows the large herniated disc lateralized to the patient's left side.

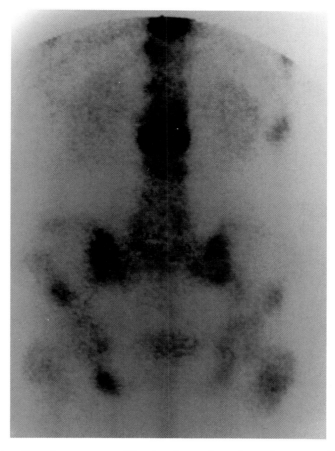

FIG. 7. A technetium bone scan of the lumbar spine shows increased uptake at L2 usually indicative of a tumor, infection, or fracture. Severe degenerative arthritis could also have this appearance. There is also some increased uptake in both sacroiliac joints, usually indicative of arthritis.

The bone scan is particularly useful for identifying areas of infection and metastatic tumor resulting in increased osteoblastic activity forming reactive sclerosis. Some tumors, however, such as multiple myeloma, may not result in increased activity on the bone scan. The bone scan may also detect trauma to bone such as osteoporotic fractures or stress fractures, which may be difficult to visualize on the CT scan or the plain radiographs. In general, the bone scan will remain "hot" for many months and sometimes over a year after an acute event such as a local fracture. The bone scan may also be useful for detecting disease in the sacroiliac joints, which can present as pain referred to the low back or buttock.

WHEN TO ORDER DIAGNOSTIC IMAGING STUDIES

The decision of when to order an imaging test is almost as important as the decision of what test to order. The vast majority of cases of acute neck pain, back pain, or radiculopathy tend to have a favorable natural history resulting in improvement with nonoperative management within 6 to 8 wk. If a neurodiagnostic imaging study is obtained too early in the course of the patient's treatment, we may obtain a picture that shows a degenerative disc or even a herniated disc. Once patients get the idea that something is broken or deranged, it is difficult for them to believe that this will resolve spontaneously, as is the case in the vast majority. So the first important message is to time the use of these expensive imaging studies judiciously because of cost effectiveness and to avoid premature disclosure to patients of clinically irrelevant information that may impede their recovery.

Accordingly, with the exception of acute trauma or the presence of a progressive neurologic deficit, most degenerative conditions should be given at least 6 wk before any aggressive imaging techniques. In fact, we recommend that plain films are not necessary for most neck and back strains, or even in cases of sciatica, for at least 4 to 6 wk. The exception to this rule would be patients who have a history that is in any way suggestive of infection or tumor, a history of prior malignancy, or age less than 20 or greater than 50. In all other cases, plain films will rarely add anything to the diagnosis at the early stage of treatment.

In the small group of patients who have been refractory to conservative management after 6 wk, the first step should generally be plain films. This will be useful to detect any gross anatomic malalignments such as spondylolisthesis as well as any signs of infection or tumor. In patients with isolated neck pain or low back pain that is refractory to appropriate nonoperative management for 4 to 6 wk and who have normal plain radiographs, the next imaging study should be a triple-phase bone scan. In cases where there is no evidence of neurologic compression and there is essentially nonradiating neck or back pain, our experience has shown that the bone scan is useful to rule out infection or tumor but can be falsely negative. In these patients without neurologic deficit or evidence of radicular pain (i.e., neck or back pain patients with referred pain), MRI or myelogram/CT scan is rarely useful at this early stage. Those studies are more useful in cases where there is a suggestion of neurologic compression. In addition, at the 6-wk point, it is helpful to obtain screening laboratory studies rather than expensive imaging studies in these patients with nonradiating low back or neck pain to rule out metabolic disease, infection, or tumor. In a patient with nonradiating low back or neck pain who has a negative work-up as described to this point, we would not recommend any more expensive techniques until nonoperative management including aggressive soft tissue and muscle rehabilitation has been attempted for a minimum of 6 mo.

In patients with evidence of nerve root or spinal cord compression, advanced imaging studies are indicated at 6 wk or earlier if there has been no clinical improvement or if there has been progression of the neurologic deficit. In younger patients with history and physical signs consistent with a herniated disc, the MR scan is probably the single most useful test. If, however, the patient is older and there is any suggestion of spinal canal stenosis, facet arthropathy, or other bone-related problems, a myelogram/CT scan may be more useful. The decision between these two tests represents a gray area and may depend on the quality of the individual tests available at the particular imaging center where one practices. Thus, blanket statements are difficult to make in this regard beyond the generalization suggested above. In rare cases, all of these tests may be necessary if there is some ambiguity that may require confirmation or localization of the most symptomatic level with a diagnostic selective nerve root block.

In the past two decades, there has been a technologic explosion in the field of neuroradiologic imaging. We have seen the development of new noninvasive techniques as well as refinement of older techniques. However, the ability to obtain better noninvasive anatomic resolution of spinal anatomy is a double-edged sword. An imaging study can be the spine surgeon's best friend or worst enemy.

Many errors in decision making with imaging studies do not come from misinterpretation of what is seen on the images; instead, they are related to how the imaging information is used and integrated into the clinical decision-making process. Because all neurodiagnostic imaging studies reveal abnormalities in at least one third of asymptomatic people, the use of these tests for general screening is dangerous. The phrase, "We'll get an MR scan to see if there is anything wrong with the spine," begins the journey down a perilous pathway. Furthermore, obtaining these expensive studies too early in the treatment of a self-limited disorder is costly and misleading, to both the physician and the patient.

When interpreting neurodiagnostic imaging studies of the spine, it is essential to have an understanding of the spectrum and frequency of abnormalities that can exist without causing symptoms. Thus, it is important to distinguish imaging abnormalities that are likely to be clinically significant from those that are part of the normal aging process. Similar problems are present on postoperative images, where it is important to distinguish true imaging abnormalities that are symptomatic from those that are part of the normal sequence of postoperative healing. The guide to making all of these distinctions must be the meticulous correlation of the anatomic location of imaging abnormalities with clinical signs and symptoms in each patient, as well as the exercise of restraint in obtaining these tests until appropriate conservative management has failed and the information obtained from the study will influence the treatment plan. Adherence to this philosophy should help avoid many of the common errors in decision making involving radiographic investigations of the spine.

SUGGESTED READING

1. Boden SD, Davis DO, Dina TS. Abnormal lumbar spine MRI scans in asymptomatic subjects: a prospective investigation. *J Bone Joint Surg [Am]*1990;72A:403–408.
2. Boden SD, McCowin PR, David DO, et al. Abnormal cervical spine MR scans in asymptomatic individuals: a prospective and blinded

investigation. *J Bone Joint Surg [Am]* 1990; 72A:1178–1184.

3. Boden SD, Wiesel SW, Laws ER, Rothman RH. *The aging spine.* Philadelphia: WB Saunders; 1991.

4. Friedenberg ZB, Miller WT. Degenerative disease of the cervical spine. *J Bone Joint Surg [Am]* 1963;45A:1171– 1178.

5. Gore DR, Sepic SB, Gardner GM. Roentgenographic findings of the cervical spine in asymptomatic people. *Spine* 1986;11:521–524.

6. Hitselberger WE, Witten RM. Abnormal myel-

ograms in asymptomatic patients. *J Neurosurg* 1968;28:204–206.

7. Shaffer WO, Spratt KT, Weinsten JN, Lehmann TR, Goel VK. The consistency and accuracy of roentgenograms for measuring sagittal translation in the lumbar vertebral motion segment: an experimental model. Volvo Award Paper. *Spine* 1990;15(8):741–750.

8. Walsh TR, Weinstein JN, Spratt KF, et al. Lumbar discography: a controlled, prospective study. *J Bone Joint Surg [Am]* 1990;72A: 1081–1088.

7

Radiologic Imaging of the Spine

Richard J. Herzog

*Department of Radiology, Hospital of the University of Pennsylvania,
Philadelphia, Pennsylvania 19104, USA*

Key Points

- The main value of plain films is to provide information about the alignment and general condition of the spine.

- Plain films give an indication of biomechanical status and the degree of the degenerative process.

- When additional information is needed, CT with multiplanar reformations and MRI are both excellent diagnostic tests.

- The strength of CT resides in its superb demonstration of osseous anatomy.

- The strength of MRI is in its excellent characterization of soft tissue abnormalities.

- In cases of spinal trauma and tumor, both CT and MRI are frequently ordered as complementary studies.

WHY ORDER AN IMAGING STUDY?

The purpose of any radiologic imaging study is to obtain morphologic information about a particular part of the body. This information is used to help solve specific clinical problems. Imaging studies may be part of the diagnostic workup of a patient or may be used to determine the effects of therapy. Before ordering any test, clinicians must ask themselves why they are ordering the test and how the information obtained from the test will affect their decision-making process. Once it is decided that additional information is needed to solve a particular clinical question or problem, the next major decision concerns the choice of the appropriate test or study to provide this information. This choice depends on the sensitivity, specificity, accuracy, risk, cost, and availability of the different studies that may be ordered. The goal of the following discussion is to provide a basic algorithm as to which radiologic examination may be of benefit in different clinical situations.

The four imaging studies most frequently ordered to evaluate spinal disorders are plain x-ray films, magnetic resonance imaging, computed tomography, and radionuclide examinations. Each test may provide useful information about specific clinical disorders. Before the selection of a test, the category of the clinical problem must be defined. This is determined by a complete history, a physical examination, and the integration of any information provided by completed diagnostic tests. The choice of which test to order next is determined by this working diagnosis. If the working diagnosis is related to the possibility of spinal infection, the appropriate test to order may be quite different than that used to evaluate radicular symptoms.

PLAIN FILMS

Even though the sensitivity and specificity of plain films in the assessment of spinal disorders is limited, they may be of benefit in determining the basic structure, integrity, and alignment of the spinal motion segments. A spinal motion segment is the combination of the discovertebral joint and the two facet joints at a specific spinal level. Whether a spinal disorder is acute or chronic can frequently be determined on plain films.

With acute disorders the pathologic changes are not associated with chronic adaptive changes (e.g., bony proliferation or endplate remodeling). Plain films are particularly important in post-traumatic conditions to evaluate spinal alignment and the integrity of the osseous structures (Fig. 1). The assessment of congenital or developmental disorders of the spine (e.g., scoliosis, transitional vertebral bodies, or developmental stenosis) that may predispose to spinal dysfunction is also provided by plain films. Plain films may be of particular benefit in patients under the age of 20 or over the age of 50 who present with back pain. In the younger patient evidence of spondylolysis or Scheuermann's disease detected on plain films may clarify the cause of back pain, and in the older patient the possibility of tumor or infection can be assessed with the standard radiographs.

In most clinical situations, plain films should be the initial imaging exam ordered in the evaluation of a spinal disorder. This does not mean that they should be ordered on every patient presenting with neck or back pain, but only when there is a specific clinical problem that must be answered. Even when it seems that additional imaging studies will be needed (e.g., MRI or CT), the plain films should still be ordered initially to provide the general information concerning the spine to which the more complex imaging studies can be correlated.

The routine plain films of the cervical and lumbar spine include anteroposterior, lateral, and oblique projections. Special coned-down lateral views

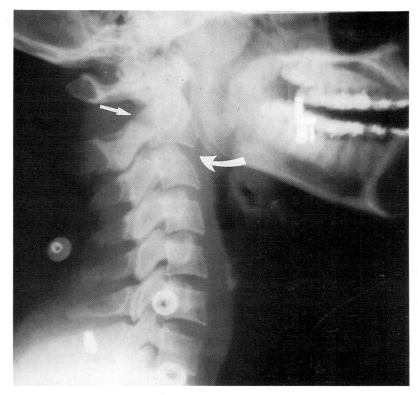

FIG. 1. Fracture of the posterior arch of C-2. On a lateral plain film of the cervical spine, there is a fracture (*straight arrow*) of the posterior arch of the C-2 vertebra, associated with a 4-mm anterolisthesis of C-2 on C-3 (*curved arrow*).

of the lumbosacral junction are also frequently obtained to evaluate the L5-S1 disc space for evidence of disc degeneration. In the cervical spine, the oblique projections are needed to evaluate post-traumatic changes and to assess the size of the neural foramina. In the lumbar spine the oblique projections are obtained to evaluate the pars interarticularis, to diagnose spondylolysis, and to evaluate the facet joints. The routine views for the thoracic spine include AP and lateral projections.

MAGNETIC RESONANCE IMAGING/COMPUTED TOMOGRAPHY

It will be assumed that one has already acquired plain films prior to ordering these additional costly studies and that they are obtained only to answer a specific diagnostic or therapeutic question.

With computed tomography, an x-ray source is used to generate cross-sectional images. Computed tomographic images are representations of differential x-ray attenuation by tissue. This attenuation is determined by the tissue's electron density. Spatial and contrast resolution is dependent on the energy of the x-ray source, slice thickness, field of view, and scanning matrix. A variety of pre- and postprocessing software programs are available to optimize the evaluation of soft tissue or osseous structures. To obtain a high-resolution multiplanar CT study, it is necessary to utilize thin (1.5 mm), contiguous sections in the cervical spine and overlapping (5 mm thick with a 2-mm overlap) or contiguous (3 mm thick) sections in the lumbar spine to create optimal computer-generated sagittal and coronal reconstructed images. The diagnostic quality of CT with multiplanar reformations (CT/MPR) is highly dependent on patient immobility to prevent misregistration artifacts. An entire CT study can currently be performed extremely quickly, particularly with the new spiral CT scanners, and, therefore, it is usually not difficult for a patient to maintain a single position. With current rapid scanning techniques, patient x-ray exposure has been significantly reduced, but still the risk of radiation exposure must be considered when ordering an examination. If a CT study is needed, a multiplanar exam should be performed, including sagittal and coronal reformations. Multiplanar CT can be obtained if the initial axial sections are contiguous or overlapping. The strength of CT is its excellent resolution of bone (Fig. 2) and, therefore, it is frequently ordered in cases of trauma to detect fractures and fracture fragment displacement. Computed tomography is also frequently obtained preoperatively in the evalua-

tion of patients with stenosis or tumors that have invaded the osseous structures.

With the implementation of high-quality MRI and CT, it is now rare that myelography or CT/myelography is needed. It still may be indicated if a diagnosis of arachnoiditis, meningeal metastasis, dural tears, pseudomeningoceles, or epidural abscess is being considered. In some centers CT-myelography is still obtained in the preoperative evaluation of patients with spinal stenosis. Radionuclide studies are usually limited to situations where screening of the entire body is required (e.g., infection or metastatic disease). Tomographic radionuclide studies may be of benefit in the detection of stress reactions or fractures of the pars interarticularis.

Whereas an image created with an x-ray source is determined by the electron density of the tissue, MR images are a construct of totally different physical properties of tissue. If a nucleus of an atom contains either unpaired protons or neutrons, it will have a net spin and angular momentum. Each spinning nucleus is surrounded by a magnetic field and can be thought of as a small bar magnet or dipole, with a north and south pole. If the body is placed in a static external magnetic field (i.e., the MR magnet), the normal random position of the nuclear dipoles in the body will be altered, and they will align themselves along the vector of the externally applied magnetic field. A magnetization vector of the tissue, which is the sum of the dipoles oriented in the same direction as the applied static magnetic field, will be created. When the spinning nuclei are aligned in the external magnetic field, they also precess (wobble) around the axis of the

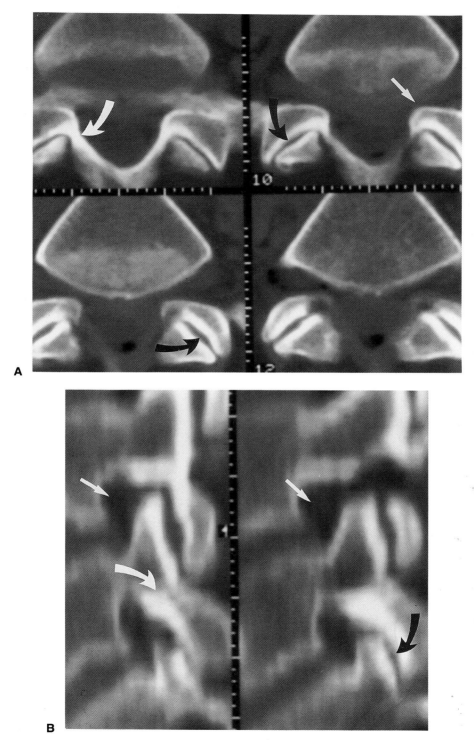

FIG. 2. Normal lumbar spine anatomy—CT/MPR-bone window. On the axial **(A)** and reformatted sagittal **(B)** CT images, there is excellent delineation of the facet joints (*curved black arrows*), neural foramina (*straight white arrow*), and pars inter-articularis (*curved white arrow*).

applied magnetic field. At present, virtually all clinical MR imaging is performed by imaging hydrogen nuclei (proton imaging). Hydrogen is an ideal atom for imaging, being the most abundant resonant nucleus in soft tissues and providing a strong MR signal.

To create an MR image, radio waves of a specific RF are pulsed into the body, which induces the transition of a fraction of the spinning protons from their equilibrium state into a higher energy state. With the termination of the RF pulse, the excited nuclei release energy and return to their lower energy state. This characteristic absorption and release of energy is called *nuclear magnetic resonance.* The transition between energy states is necessary for the construction of an MR image. The process of returning from the excited to the equilibrium state is called *relaxation* and is characterized by two independent time constants, T1 and T2. The T1 (longitudinal relaxation time) reflects the time required for excited protons to return to their equilibrium state. When the hydrogen nucleus is excited by the application of an RF pulse, in addition to changing to a higher energy state the initially random precession of the nuclei prior to excitation will become coherent (in phase) after excitation. This results in a magnetization vector perpendicular (transverse) to the external magnetic field, which can be directly measured by a receiver coil. With the termination of the RF pulse, there is rapid loss of coherence of the precessing nuclei, and the T2 (transverse relaxation time) is the time reflecting the loss of the transverse magnetization.

T1 and T2 relaxation are intrinsic physical properties of tissue. The MR signal intensity is mainly dependent on the T1, T2, and proton density (number of mobile hydrogen ions) of the tissue being evaluated. To obtain an anatomic image, spatial encoding of the energy released by the excited protons must be performed in three anatomic planes. This is accomplished by creating small gradient magnetic fields within the larger static applied field. The methods for obtaining MR data are designated *pulse sequences.* Spin echo (SE) and gradient echo (GE) are currently the pulse sequences most often employed. The spin-echo pulse sequence is probably the most commonly used MRI sequence, and the images created are dependent upon several scanning parameters. The repetition time (TR—the time between RF pulses) and the echo time (TE—the time between the application of the RF pulse and the recording the MR signal) are determined before acquiring the image. By varying the scanning parameters (TR and TE), the relative contribution of the T1, T2, and proton density of the tissue will determine image contrast. A *T1-weighted image,* which emphasizes the T1 properties of a tissue, is produced with a short TR (400 to 600 ms) and a short TE (15 to 30 ms). T1-weighted images are ideal for evaluating structures containing fat, subacute or chronic hemorrhage, or proteinaceous fluid because these materials have a short T1 and yield a high signal on T1-weighted sequences. T1-weighted images, frequently thought of as fat images, are excellent in the delineation of anatomic structures. An MR image produced with a long TR (1,500 to 2,000 ms) and a short TE (15 to 30 ms) is referred to as a *pro-*

ton-density or *spin-density weighted image,* and the signal intensity reflects the absolute number of mobile hydrogen ions in the tissue. A *T2-weighted sequence,* which emphasizes the T2 properties of tissue, requires a long TR (1,500 to 3,000 ms) and a long TE (60 to 120 ms). The signal intensity on T2-weighted images is related to the state of hydration of the tissue. Any tissue rich in free or extracellular water (e.g., cerebrospinal fluid, cysts, necrotic tissue, fluid collections, intervertebral discs, and neoplasms) will demonstrate increased signal intensity on T2-weighted sequences. Mineral-rich tissue (e.g., bone) contains few mobile protons and consequently demonstrates very low signal intensity on all pulse sequences. Gas, containing no mobile hydrogen ions, generates no MR signal.

In addition to signal intensity, tissue and organ configuration must be evaluated to detect pathologic changes. Spatial resolution, the ability to delineate fine detail, is determined by slice thickness, field of view (FOV), and the size of the acquisition and display matrices. Ideally, when imaging small structures, thin sections with a large matrix (256 x 256 or 512 x 512) should be utilized, but MRI, like CT, is affected by signal-to-noise constraints, and image degradation may result from low signal-to-noise ratios. Improved spatial resolution on MRI evaluations can be achieved by using surface coils, with their higher signal-to-noise ratio, but at the cost of a smaller field of view.

As in all imaging procedures, artifacts are a source of image degradation in MRI studies, resulting in significant loss of diagnostic information. Motion artifacts are the most common cause of image degradation. In CT studies patient motion results in the degradation of a single image, but movement during MRI scanning will cause degradation of all images in a sequence. To decrease scan time, new fast-scanning methods have been developed (e.g., fast spin-echo imaging and gradient echo imaging). With gradient echo imaging, gradient reversal is used to restore the transverse magnetization vector in order to generate an MR signal, instead of using an additional radiofrequency (RF) pulse, which is utilized with spin-echo imaging. There is a wide range of potential image contrast using gradient echo imaging by manipulating its repetition time (TR), echo time (TE), and flip angle. The contrast obtained with gradient echo imaging is referred to as $T2^*$ (T2 star) and is different from the standard T2 contrast obtained on spin-echo sequences. Potential degradation of gradient echo imaging due to magnetic field inhomogeneities is greater than with spin-echo imaging. The information obtained from gradient echo sequences is different from standard T1- and T2-weighted sequences, and it cannot be considered a simple replacement for a standard spin-echo sequence.

Standard MRI studies of the spine include sagittal spin-echo T1- and T2-weighted sequences along with a spin-echo T1-weighted axial sequence (Fig. 3). Gradient echo $T2^*$ axial and sagittal sequences are also frequently obtained. In the cervical spine thinner sections are needed compared to the lumbar spine because of the smaller size of the anatomic structures. The strength of MRI resides in its excellent soft tissue contrast, direct

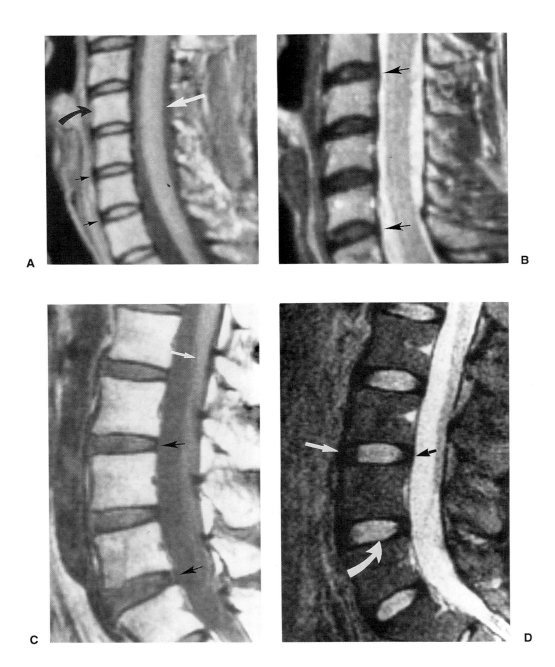

multiplanar imaging, and absence of ionizing radiation. The major contraindication to an MRI study is the presence of any electrical device in the body (e.g., a cardiac pacemaker or medication pump), brain aneurysm clips, some cochlear and ocular implants, some vascular filters, and metallic fragments in the eye or spinal canal. Patients with claustrophobia may have difficulty with the performance of the exam, but they usually can complete the study if they receive information about the study before undergoing the exam. Medications can also be provided to relieve anxiety, if needed. For evaluation of the traumatized patient, MRI-compatible spine stabilizers and support equipment are now available.

The most common clinical conditions involving the spinal column that require diagnostic evaluation are degenerative spinal disease (which includes disc and facet degeneration along with spinal stenosis), postoperative disorders, spinal trauma, metastatic disease, spondyloarthropathies, and spinal infection.

DEGENERATIVE DISC DISEASE

When trying to understand the dynamic changes that are identified in the degenerating spine, it is helpful to think of each disc level in the spine as a motion segment or a functional unit comprising the discovertebral joint and the two facet joints. It is important to evaluate all components of this functional unit with imaging studies and not merely to focus on isolated pathologic changes (e.g., disc herniation).

For the evaluation of disc degeneration, plain films are of limited value. Decreased disc height, bony sclerosis, gas or calcification within the disc space, and endplate hyperostosis are associated with degenerative changes of the disc, but these findings are of little predictive

---

FIG. 3. Normal spine anatomy—MRI. On the sagittal T1-weighted image **(A)** of the cervical spine, there is excellent demonstration of the cervical spinal cord (*straight white arrow),* the vertebral bodies (*curved black arrow),* and the discovertebral joint (*short black arrow*). On the sagittal T2-weighted image **(B)**, there is high signal intensity within the cerebrospinal fluid surrounding the spinal cord, which results in excellent delineation of the margins of the spinal cord and optimal evaluation of the posterior margin of the discovertebral joints (*black arrows*). On the sagittal T1-weighted image of the lumbar spine **(C)**, there is excellent delineation of the conus medullaris (*white arrow*). The intervertebral disc space is well delineated, but the posterior margin of the disc is not well defined because of the similar signal intensity of the posterior outer annular fibers and the adjacent cerebrospinal fluid (*black arrows*). On the sagittal T2-weighted image **(D)**, there is increased signal intensity within the cerebrospinal fluid and excellent delineation of the posterior margin of the disc (*black arrow*). There is increased signal intensity within the central portion of the disc (*curved white arrow*), which represents a combination of the nucleus pulposus and the inner annular fibers. The anterior annular fibers (*straight white arrow*) are also delineated.

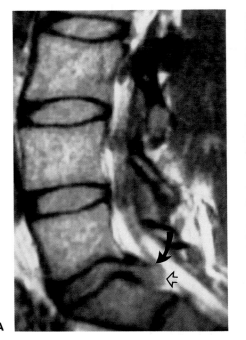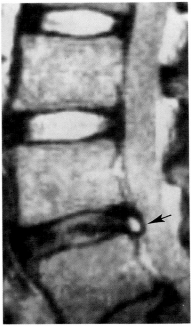

A   **B**

FIG. 4. Lumbar spine disc extrusion and protrusion. At the L5-S1 disc level, on the sagittal proton-density weighted image **(A)**, there is a posterior disc extrusion (*open black arrow*) that has penetrated through the posterior outer annular-posterior longitudinal ligament complex (*curved arrow*). On another patient, on the sagittal T2-weighted image **(B)**, there is a posterior disc protrusion (*arrow*) contained by the posterior outer annular-posterior longitudinal ligament complex.

value in determining the cause of spinal or radicular pain. For the evaluation of disc disease, both MRI and CT provide excellent delineation of disc herniation. The major difference between the imaging techniques is that MRI can detect pathoanatomic and chemical changes within the disc prior to changes in disc contour. On an MRI spin-echo T2-weighted sequence, the signal intensity of the disc is related to the state of hydration of the nucleus pulposus and the inner annular fibers. With aging and degeneration there is gradual desiccation of the mucoid nuclear material and transfor-

mation of the disc into a more solid fibrocartilaginous structure. With desiccation and degeneration of the disc, there will be loss of the high signal intensity in the disc on the T2-weighted images. The development of a radial annular tear is probably the necessary step in the development of a disc herniation. With MRI, it is possible to delineate these tears before the displacement of nuclear material (i.e., disc herniation). Displacement of nuclear material into the region of the outer annular fibers will cause a focal contour abnormality of the disc (i.e., a *disc protrusion*). As long as the disc material is contained by the outer annulus or the posterior longitudinal ligament, it is considered a contained herniation. If it penetrates the outer annular-posterior long-itudinal ligament complex, it is called a *disc extrusion* (Fig. 4). If the disc material separates from its disc of origin, it is called a *sequestered fragment.* This fragment may migrate cranial or caudal to the disc space. Both CT and MRI are excellent techniques to detect and characterize disc herniations. After a disc has herniated, the disc material within the disc space will continue to degenerate and on an MRI study the degenerated disc will demonstrate low signal intensity on spin-echo T2-weighted images. There may be fluid-filled fissures and granulation tissue within the degenerated disc, which are detected as foci of high signal intensity on T2-weighted images. This should not be confused with an inflammatory process. Endplate degeneration is frequently associated with disc degeneration. These changes can be detected on the MRI study as areas of abnormal signal intensity in the subchondral bone; these areas reflect the presence of fibrovascular tissue or fatty infiltration. Bony sclerosis or proliferation can be detected with CT or plain films. With the increased utilization of MRI, it has become clear that degenerative disc disease is a process that often begins in the second or third decade and progresses as an individual ages. Evidence of a disc herniation or disc degeneration is frequently identified on imaging studies, in both symptomatic and asymptomatic individuals. The significance of these findings can be determined only by precise correlation to the clinical findings.

With disc degeneration there is alteration of the biomechanical status of the functional unit, which may precipitate degenerative changes in the facet joints. Degenerative changes of the facet joints include cartilage erosion, subchondral cysts, bony sclerosis, and osteophyte formation. Both CT and MRI can detect these degenerative changes, but only MRI can delineate changes of the articular cartilage and demonstrate joint effusions. Plain films are much less sensitive in detecting early degenerative changes of the facet joints.

SPINAL STENOSIS

Spinal stenosis is a local, segmental, or generalized narrowing of the central spinal canal, the lateral recesses, or the neural foramina by bony or soft tissue elements. The resultant narrowing may encroach upon the neural structures. The degenerative changes that most commonly cause stenosis include osteophytes of the vertebral body endplates, uncinate processes, or facet joints and hypertrophy of the ligamenta flava and anterior facet capsule. The initial size of the spinal canal is an important factor in determining whether degenerative changes will cause neural impingement or compression. The role of both CT and MRI is accurately to delineate the nature and extent of stenosis and to define which of the degenerative elements is the cause of the stenotic process.

The initial examination in the evaluation of a patient with cervical radiculopathy or myelopathy, after obtaining plain films, is an MRI. The strength of MRI is its ability to evaluate the entire

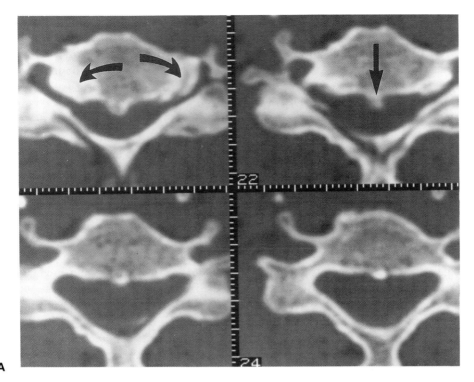

A

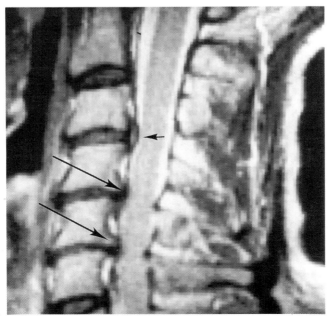

B

cervical spine completely, including the discovertebral joint and the spinal cord (Fig. 5). The major limitation of MRI in the past was in the assessment of the neural foramina. Currently, however, with the thinner sections and the ability to acquire direct oblique images through the neural foramina, the MRI exam provides an excellent complete study. Occasionally CT is ordered to evaluate further the osseous contributions to the stenotic process. With patients presenting with myelopathy, it is important to determine the accurate size of the central spinal canal. Only on a midline sagittal image is it possible to measure the degree of developmental central canal stenosis. Osseous stenosis does not necessarily cause cervical myelopathy, and the strength of MRI is its ability to determine the effect of the degenerative processes on the neural elements, particularly the spinal cord. Patients presenting with myelopathic symptoms frequently have degenerative spondylotic changes superimposed on a developmentally small canal. The best predictor of the clinical course in myelopathic patients has been MRI studies. High signal intensity within the cord on T2-weighted sequences and decreased cord volume seem to indicate a poorer prognosis for these patients whether they undergo operative or nonoperative therapy. Because CT-myelography is an invasive procedure, it is ordered only when the other studies are not adequate or contraindicated.

Cervical radiculopathy is usually secondary to a posterolateral disc herniation or nerve root impingement in the neural foramen secondary to degenerative changes of the uncovertebral joints. Both CT and MRI can be utilized in the evaluation of radicular symptoms. Magnetic resonance imaging is optimal for the detection of disc material, whereas CT is optimal to determine the degree of osseous stenosis. Magnetic resonance imaging is usually ordered before CT because it provides a complete evaluation of the entire cervical spine and it does not use ionizing radiation. If there is a contraindication for an MRI study, then CT is routinely obtained. The addition of multiplanar reformations to a CT study is important to provide the maximal amount of information concerning the pathologic changes.

In the assessment of lumbar spinal stenosis, it is helpful to determine the type of stenosis present (e.g., developmental or acquired). *Developmental*

FIG. 5. Stenosis of the cervical central spinal canal and neural foramina. The axial CT **(A)** was obtained to determine the degree of stenosis of the neural foramina (*curved black arrows*). A bone ridge (*straight black arrow*) is also identified projecting off the posterior margin of the vertebral body. The MRI study is optimal to evaluate the central spinal canal, particularly the effects of cervical spondylosis on the spinal cord. On the MRI sagittal T2-weighted image **(B)**, a posterior disc protrusion at the C3-4 disc level is causing minimal cord impingement (*short black arrow*). Changes of cervical spondylosis are present at the C4-5 and C5-6 levels with spondylotic ridges (*long black arrows*) causing mild cord impingement. The signal intensity within the spinal cord is normal.

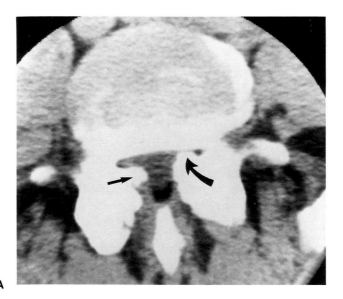

FIG. 6. Central canal stenosis at the L4-5 disc level. On the axial CT images (**A** and **B**), there are severe degenerative changes of the facet joints with prominent osteophytes causing stenosis of the subarticular and lateral recesses and the central spinal canal. The proliferative changes of the left facet joint (*curved black arrow*) are causing severe stenosis of the left subarticular lateral recess, and the proliferative changes of the right facet joint (*straight black arrow*) are causing moderate stenosis.

stenosis is a growth disturbance of the posterior elements involving the pedicles, laminae, and facet joints. This results in decreased volume of the central spinal canal or neural foramina, which may predispose to neural impingement. A midline sagittal diameter of less than 12 mm is considered *relative stenosis,* and a diameter of less than 10 mm is considered *absolute stenosis.* This diameter is measured from the middle of the posterior surface of the vertebral body to the junction point of the base of the spinous process and the laminae. This same measurement can be performed in the cervical spine.

Acquired stenosis is the narrowing of the central spinal canal or the neural foramina by degenerative changes of the discovertebral joints, facet joints, and ligamenta flava. Both CT and MRI can accurately assess the degree of central canal narrowing. Before performing a decompressive procedure for stenosis of the central spinal canal or the lateral recesses, it is necessary to define precisely the location and extent of the degenerative elements that are encroaching on the neural elements so that an adequate decompression can be achieved. It is also important not to remove any structures that are not contributing to the patient's symptoms, thereby decreasing the chance of postoperative instability. The strength of CT is its ability to demonstrate osseous proliferative changes that may be narrowing the subarticular and lateral recesses (Fig. 6). The strength of MRI is that it provides the ability to measure noninvasively the cross-sectional area of the thecal sac, which in some clinical studies has the best correlation to the patient's stenotic symptoms. Before the development and implementation of MRI, a myelogram or CT-myelogram was needed to determine the degree of narrowing of the thecal sac.

Foraminal stenosis is an important cause of radicular symptoms and, if it is not corrected at the time of surgery, it is a frequent cause of failed back surgery. Each neural foramen is actually a short canal with an entrance, middle, and exit zone. The length of the canal increases at the lower lumbar motion segments as a result of the wider pedicles, and at the L5-S1 disc level the canal may measure 12 mm long. Degenerative ridges projecting off the posterolateral margin of the vertebral body endplates may narrow the entrance, middle, or exit zone, and the exact location of the stenosis must be determined if surgery is undertaken (Fig. 7). The size and location of these ridges will determine the operative approach and the amount of bone that must be removed to decompress the neural elements. Facet degenerative changes may also narrow the neural foramina, in addition to narrowing the central spinal canal and lateral recesses. In elderly patients with scoliosis and in patients with isthmic spondylolisthesis, there may be compression of the L5 nerve root after it exits the neural foramen (i.e., far-out or extraforaminal stenosis). This neural compression occurs between the base of the L5 transverse process and the sacral ala.

Degenerative spondylolisthesis is an important potential cause of central canal and foraminal stenosis. This most frequently is identified in middle-aged or elderly individuals and involves the L4-5 disc level. It is the result of degen-

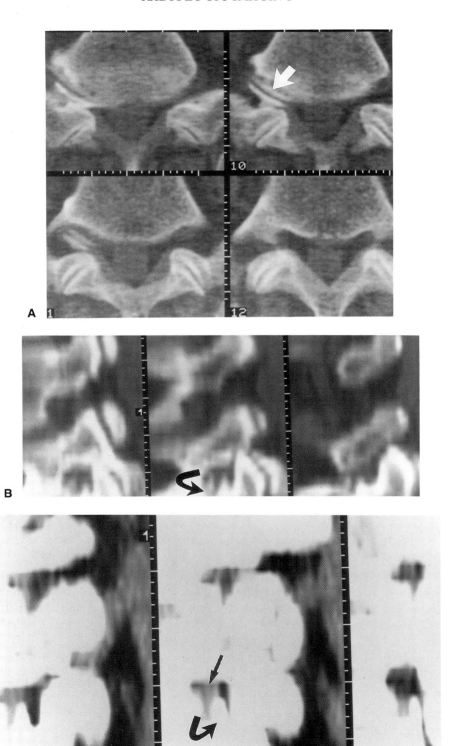

erative changes of the disc and the facet joints and a secondary anterolisthesis. Sagittally oriented facet joints predispose to anterolisthesis, and both MRI and CT can be used to assess the orientation and associated degenerative changes of the facet joints. With a degenerative spondylolisthesis the anterolisthesis rarely progresses beyond Grade 1 because of the intact neural arch. The stenosis of the central canal is secondary to the proliferative changes of the anteromedial margins of the facet joints, hypertrophy of the ligamenta flava, posterior annular redundancy, and the anterolisthesis. Stenosis of the subarticular and lateral recesses is also frequently identified with these degenerative changes.

SPINAL TRAUMA

Traumatic spinal disorders are secondary to chronic microtrauma as well as acute macrotrauma. The initial evaluation of patients presenting with a history of trauma includes routine plain film studies, which are sometimes followed by flexion and extension films to assess spinal alignment and stability. The severity and extent of the injury will determine the type of films that are ordered.

Isthmic spondylolysis usually represents a stress fracture of the pars interarticularis, which is related to chronic overloading of the pars in the adolescent.

Occasionally the fracture may be secondary to an acute extension injury related to athletics or other forms of acute spinal trauma (e.g., a motor vehicle injury). Fracture of the pars may precipitate back pain but also is frequently detected in asymptomatic individuals. Tomographic radionuclide studies are probably the most sensitive test to detect stress reactions and early stress fractures of the pars. Before a complete stress fracture, evidence of increased bone turnover may be detected on a tomographic radionuclide study. These stress reactions have been associated with the onset of back pain. After the fracture has been present for a short time, there will be bone resorption or hypertrophy at the fracture site, and multiplanar CT is the optimal test to delineate the structural changes (Fig. 8). Fragmentation and hypertrophy of the pars interarticularis can cause stenosis of the central spinal canal or the neural foramina. The fracture of the pars is usually bilateral and most often involves the L-5 vertebra. If there is an anterior displacement of the L-5 vertebral body with respect to the S-1 vertebral body, the malalignment is called a *spondylolisthesis*. The degree of anterolisthesis is usually classified as Grade 1 to 4 depending on the degree of anterior displacement of the L-5 vertebral body with respect to the S-1 vertebral body. A Grade 1 spondylolisthesis

FIG. 7. Lumbar foraminal stenosis. On the axial CT image **(A)**, osseous ridges (*white arrow*) project into the right neural foramen. On the sagittal reformatted images (**B** and **C**), the narrowing of the neural foramen at the L5-S1 disc level by the osseous ridges (*curved black arrow*), along with the compression of the exiting left L5 nerve root (*straight black arrow*) are identified.

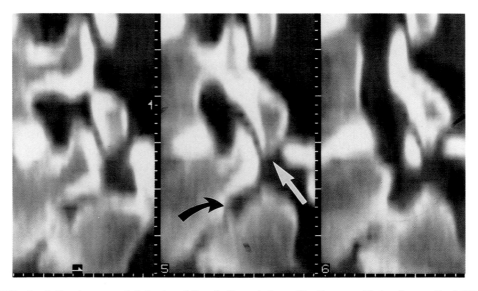

FIG. 8. Isthmic spondylolysis of the L-5 vertebra. On the sagittal reformatted CT image, there is excellent delineation of the defect in the pars interarticularis (*straight arrow*). There is severe stenosis of the neural foramen (*curved arrow*) secondary to the anterolisthesis and the decreased disc height.

is present if the L-5 vertebral body is displaced anteriorly less than 25% the length of the superior surface of the S-1 vertebral body. The higher grades represent further anterior displacement of L-5, with each grade representing one quarter of the length of the superior surface of the S-1 vertebral body. Erect films should be obtained to determine the degree of anterolisthesis. Flexion and extension films are also useful to demonstrate whether there is abnormal spinal motion related to the spondylolysis or spondylolisthesis. Patients with spondylolysis have an increased incidence of disc degeneration and herniation at the level of the spondylolysis and at the adjacent disc level. This may be the cause of the patient's symptoms and can be determined on the MRI or CT study. One

major limitation of the radionuclide study in the assessment of spondylolysis is that it can detect only the osseous abnormalities and cannot demonstrate the discal abnormality nor determine whether stenosis is present.

Symptoms related to acute macrotrauma to the spine are usually related to injuries of the cervical spine or the thoracolumbar junction. The optimal treatment of cervical cord injury secondary to vertebral fractures and subluxation is still evolving. The evaluation of patients with a cervical spine injury includes AP and lateral views of the spine along with an open-mouth view of the odontoid. On the lateral view it is necessary to visualize from the occipitocervical junction to the C7-T1 disc level. If this cannot be achieved on the routine lateral projection, then additional special views should be performed (e.g., a swimmer's view to visualize the C7-T1 motion segment). In adults, if the space between the anterior arch of C-1 and the odontoid is greater than 3 mm or if there is a 3 mm anterior or posterior translation of one vertebral body on another, the patient must be further evaluated and treated for the possibility of instability. Other signs of instability (e.g., fracture type and abnormal vertebral angular alignment) must also be assessed at the time of injury. Flexion and extension films are needed to detect motion abnormalities of the spine (e.g., hypermobile or hypomobile motion segments). During the immediate post-traumatic period, these studies may be difficult to perform because of neck pain, and the patient must return for further evaluation of spinal stability when he is free of pain. With MRI it is now possible to evaluate spinal cord injuries directly by detecting edematous and hemorrhagic changes within the cord. Several recent clinical series have suggested that the presence of blood in the cord is a poor prognostic indicator, whereas the chance for complete recovery is significantly greater if only edematous changes are identified on the MRI study. The occipitocervical junction and the C1-2 motion segment can also be evaluated on an MRI study. It is possible to perform a supervised MRI study with the patient's neck in flexion and extension to determine the stability of the cervical motion segments.

CT with multiplanar reformations is still the optimal study to detect fractures, particularly of the posterior elements. The roles of CT and MRI are frequently complementary, and often both studies are obtained to evaluate pathologic changes. This is particularly true at the thoracolumbar junction, where MRI is needed to determine the position of the conus medullaris and to detect a conus injury, whereas CT is needed to evaluate the position of the fracture fragments and to determine the degree of central canal compromise (Fig. 9). In the follow-up evaluation of a traumatized patient, MRI is optimal to detect post-traumatic cysts or myelomalacia and CT may be needed to determine the degree of fracture healing and bone remodeling.

POSTOPERATIVE EVALUATION OF THE SPINE

In several clinical situations patients who have undergone spinal surgery may need repeat evaluation with diagnostic imaging studies. It is not infrequent for patients to experience persistent or recurrent back pain after spinal surgery, and the differential diagnostic possibilities as to potential causes of patient symptoms include central canal or foraminal stenosis, disc herniation, arachnoiditis, epidural fibrosis, nerve injury, and infection. The reason for the initial surgery and the type of surgical procedure that was performed will frequently direct the work-up of the patient's dysfunction.

If a patient has had prior disc surgery and presents with persistent or recurrent symptoms, an MRI exam is the optimal method to detect the presence of discal abnormality. The interval between the surgery and the MRI exam is important because the specificity of the study is limited in the first 6 mo after surgery. In this initial 6-mo period, it is extremely

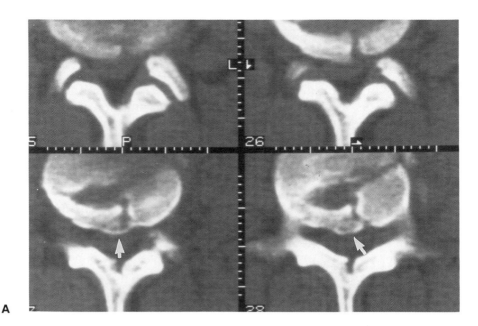

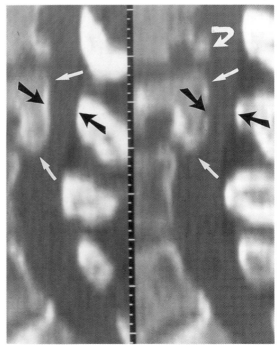

FIG. 9. Post-traumatic central canal stenosis. On the axial CT image **(A)**, the fracture deformity of the inferior endplate of L-2 is identified, with dorsal displacement of the posterior segment of the vertebral body resulting in stenosis of the central spinal canal (*arrows*). The reformatted sagittal CT image **(B)** is optimal to demonstrate the retropulsion of the endplate fracture (*curved white arrow*). In addition, there is a post-traumatic deformity of the L-3 vertebral body with posterior displacement of the vertebral body (*straight white arrows*). The degree of stenosis is greatest posterior to the midbody of L-3 (*straight black arrows*).

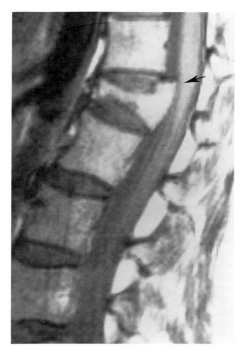

C

FIG. 9. *(Continued)*. On another patient, on the sagittal T1-weighted MR image **(C)**, there is a compression fracture of the L-1 vertebral body with retropulsion of the compressed vertebral body resulting in minimal impingement of the conus medullaris (*arrow*).

common to identify abnormal morphology of the posterior margin of the disc in asymptomatic patients. After this period, the MRI study provides a complete evaluation of the operative level by being able to detect abnormal disc material and separate it from postoperative fibrotic changes (Fig. 10). The study is routinely performed with and without the injection of a contrast agent (e.g., gadolinium-DTPA), which enhances the fibrotic material. There have been few adverse side effects related to the administration of gadolinium-DTPA (diethylene triamine pentaacetic acid).

Patients with the failed back surgery syndrome present with a variety of postoperative findings. Epidural fibrosis is frequently present at the operative site and typically demonstrates intermediate signal intensity on an MRI T1-weighted image and increased signal intensity on a T2-weighted image. Fibrosis is usually poorly marginated and typically generates little mass effect. Recurrent disc herniations are usually contiguous with the disc space, are well marginated, and, when compared to the disc of origin, demonstrate isointensity or hypointensity on a T1-weighted sequence and isointensity or hyperintensity on a T2-weighted sequence. With MRI it is also possible to detect the other possible causes of pain in these patients, including foraminal stenosis, arachnoiditis, disc infection, epidural abscess, and pseudo-meningoceles.

In patients who have had a decompressive procedure to correct spinal stenosis and who present with recurrent symptoms of stenosis, it is necessary to evaluate the degree of osseous regrowth and the presence of residual or recurrent stenosis. It is also important to determine whether there is evidence of instability secondary to the prior surgical procedure. Both CT and MRI provide useful information in the evaluation of these patients. Computed tomography is the optimal study to evaluate the degree of osseous stenosis, and it is particularly helpful in the evaluation of the subarticular lateral recess. With MRI it is possible to determine the degree of thecal sac compression at the stenotic level. Both CT with

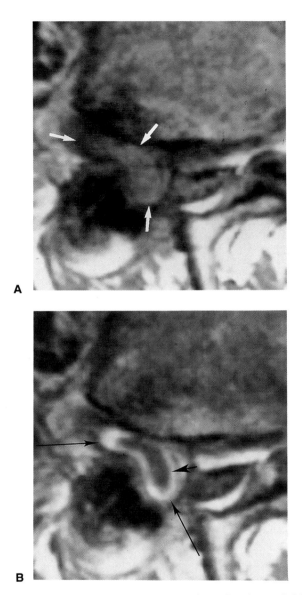

FIG. 10. Postoperative recurrent disc herniation. On the axial T1-weighted MR image **(A)**, a large soft tissue extradural mass (*arrows*) is present compressing the right side of the thecal sac and extending into the right neural foramen. After the administration of gadolinium-DTPA, a repeat axial T1-weighted image **(B)** demonstrates a large disc fragment (*short black arrow*) surrounded by a bright band of fibrotic material (*long black arrows*).

multiplanar reformations and MRI are excellent in assessing the degree of foraminal stenosis.

When a fusion has been performed for spinal stabilization, the question of the status of the fusion arises if the patient develops recurrent symptoms. The sensitivity and specificity of plain films, including flexion and extension views, are poor in detecting the presence of a pseudarthrosis. The status of a fusion is optimally evaluated with a multiplanar CT study. Reformatted images in both the coronal and the sagittal plane are needed to assess the solidity of a fusion mass. This is particularly true in the assessment of posterolateral or intertransverse process fusions. Both CT and MRI can be used to evaluate an interbody fusion. Continuous bone bridging must be demonstrated to diagnose a solid fusion.

Occasionally the question of infection arises during the postoperative period. An MRI study utilizing gadolinium-DTPA is the optimal screening study for these patients. Radionuclide studies lack the specificity and the spatial resolution provided by the MRI examination. In some cases it also may be necessary to obtain a CT-myelogram if the MRI results are inconclusive and there is a clinical suspicion of an epidural abscess.

If posterior instrumentation has been performed as part of the operative procedure, both the CT and the MRI studies will usually demonstrate some type of image degradation secondary to the implanted metal. The size, position, orientation, and composition of the instrumentation determine the extent of the artifact. Most metallic constructs gener-

ate a large amount of artifact on an MRI study unless it is composed of nonferromagnetic material such as titanium. Artifacts are also a problem on a CT exam, particularly if the area of interest is at the level of pedicular screws. Computed tomography will usually provide more information than will MRI in the assessment of these patients.

SPINAL TUMORS

Patients with primary or metastatic tumors involving the spinal cord or the vertebral column may present with a rapidly progressive myelopathy, myeloradiculopathy, or radiculopathy, but most frequently their symptoms are subacute or chronic. Plain films should be the first imaging study obtained, even though they are insensitive for the detection of osseous metastases. Approximately 40% to 50% of the cancellous bone of the vertebral body must be destroyed before an abnormality will be detected on plain films. Frequently, one can detect the destruction of a pedicle before the destruction of the vertebral body because the pedicle contains a higher percentage of cortical bone. The main value of the plain film is in detecting a fracture or malalignment of the spinal column secondary to the infiltrative process.

MRI is the optimal examination in the evaluation of patients for a suspected tumor. Tumors may be localized to different compartments of the neuraxis and are classified as (a) intramedullary, (b) intradural-extramedullary, (c) extradural, and (d) osseous. Some tumors may be found in two locations, and this is a typical presentation of metastatic disease.

With MRI it is possible to evaluate all potential sites of tumor involvement, and MRI is particularly sensitive to any process invading or destroying the cancellous bone of the vertebra and extending into the central spinal canal or the paravertebral soft tissue. With the aid of gadolinium-DTPA, it is possible to separate viable from necrotic tissue if a biopsy is needed. With an intraspinal tumor both the morphology and the signal intensity of the spinal cord may be abnormal on the MRI study. Osseous metastatic deposits to the vertebral marrow are detected by abnormal signal intensity in the bone marrow on spin-echo or short-tau inversion recovery (STIR) sequences. STIR sequences are extremely sensitive to any process that increases the fluid content in the cancellous bone. It is important to realize that these abnormal findings are not specific for metastatic tumor but are also identified in any pathologic process causing increased fluid in the cancellous bone (e.g., infection or edema after a vertebral fracture). Radionuclide studies are frequently obtained if the entire skeleton is

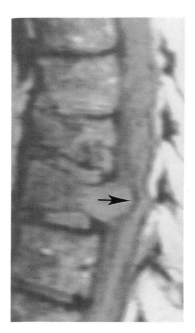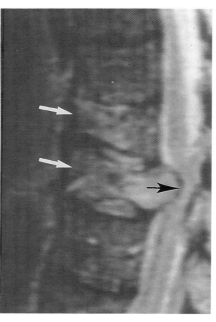

A   **B**

FIG. 11. Multiple myeloma. On the sagittal T1-weighted MR image **(A)**, there is a compressed and deformed T-12 vertebral body. Dorsal displacement of the vertebral body is causing severe stenosis (*arrow*) of the central spinal canal. On the sagittal T2-weighted image **(B)**, there is increased signal intensity in the T-11 and T-12 vertebral bodies (*white arrows*), secondary to the myelomatous deposits. With the increased signal intensity in the cerebrospinal fluid, the degree of central canal stenosis and cord compression is optimally delineated (*straight black arrow*).

being evaluated for the presence of metastatic disease. The sensitivities of MRI and radionuclide studies are similar except with multiple myeloma, where MRI is more sensitive. The value of MRI is its superior spatial resolution compared to the radionuclide exam (Fig 11).

The value of CT is in the assessment of the degree of osseous destruction, which may help determine the risk of a fracture. A CT study may be obtained before a surgical procedure to demonstrate the extent of osseous involvement, particularly if a decompression and stabilization procedure is being considered. Computed tomography-myelography is occasionally performed in the preoperative evaluation of these patients if the routine noninvasive studies are not adequate.

SPINAL INFECTION

Spinal infection in the adult typically involves the disc space and the contiguous vertebral bodies. The source of the infection is usually secondary to hematogenous seeding from a remote site, frequently from the genitourinary system in the older patient. The infection begins in the vertebral endplate and spreads to the adjacent disc and vertebral body. This is characteristic of most pyogenic agents. With tuberculosis and some other granulomatous infective agents, the inflammatory focus may remain in the vertebral body or extend into the paravertebral soft tissue and not involve the adjacent disc. If a surgical procedure has been performed on the disc, an infection may be initially localized to the disc space, thus representing a true discitis. The infection may then spread to the adja-

cent vertebral bodies. Primary discitis may occur in young children when the vascular supply to the outer margins of their discs is still intact.

MRI should be the initial screening exam in the evaluation of a patient for spinal infection. The findings on an MRI study include the following: (a) on a sagittal T1-weighted image, there is confluent decreased signal intensity in the vertebral bodies and intervertebral disc; (b) on a sagittal T2-weighted image, there is increased signal intensity in the disc and the vertebral bodies and poor delineation of the vertebral body endplates; and (c) there are inflammatory changes in the paravertebral soft tissues (Fig. 12). The sensitivity, specificity, and accuracy of MRI are comparable to those of the combination of a bone scan and a gallium study. The major advantages of an MRI study is that it provides excellent visualization of the spinal cord and the central spinal canal and can determine whether the inflammatory process extends beyond the margins of the disc and bone. With an MRI, it is also possible to detect the presence of a focal abscess. The MRI findings of nonpyogenic osteomyelitis may be atypical, suggesting a neoplasm rather than an infection. Tuberculous spondylitis may present as focal involvement of the vertebral body or posterior elements. Magnetic resonance imaging studies utilizing gadolinium-DTPA should be performed initially for the evaluation of an epidural abscess. If the findings on an MRI study are inconclusive, a CT-myelogram may of value.

Occasionally a patient who is undergoing treatment for a spinal infection will need to be re-evaluated to determine

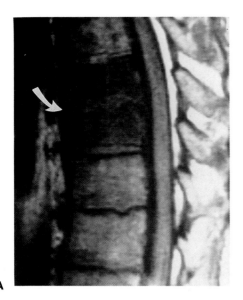 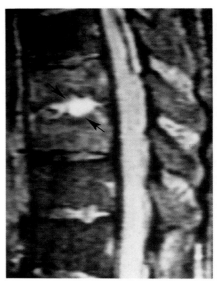

A **B**

FIG. 12. Pyogenic vertebral osteomyelitis. On the MRI sagittal T1-weighted image **(A)**, there is a confluent area of decreased signal intensity in the T-7 and T-8 vertebral bodies and the intervening disc (*arrow*). On the sagittal T2-weighted image **(B)**, there is increased signal intensity in the disc space (*arrows*), along with diffuse increased signal intensity in the adjacent vertebral bodies.

whether there is evidence of healing of the inflammatory focus. Magnetic resonance imaging utilizing gadolinium-DTPA has been useful in the evaluation of these patients. Frequently the abnormal appearance of the disc space lags behind the clinical improvement of the patient. In a small series of cases, MRI with gadolinium-DTPA was also helpful in separating infectious from noninfectious discitis during the immediate postoperative period.

SPONDYLOARTHROPATHIES

Because the spine is a composite of amphiarthroses, diarthroses, and entheses, it may be affected by a variety of arthritic processes. Usually, routine plain films are adequate to evaluate patients with arthritic symptoms if one realizes that they are not sensitive in the detection of early disease. Flexion and extension films are helpful in the evaluation of instability in patients with rheumatoid arthritis involving the cervical spine. Patients with longstanding rheumatoid arthritis may develop erosions of the odontoid process and destruction of the transverse ligament of C-2 by proliferation of pannus, which results in instability at the C1-2 motion segment. They also may develop cranial migration of the dens or subaxial subluxation. Magnetic resonance imaging has been particularly helpful in the evaluation of rheumatoid patients who present with symptoms of myelopathy or myeloradiculopathy. With MRI it is possible to demonstrate whether there is cord compression by pannus or as a result of osseous malalignment. Magnetic resonance studies in flexion and extension can also be performed to determine the stability of an abnormal motion segment.

In the lumbar spine, degenerative joint disease frequently affects the facet joints at levels with disc degeneration. At the L4-5 disc level, degenerative facet disease may precipitate an anterolisthesis, particularly if the facets have a sagittal orientation. In addition to the routine plain films, flexion and extension films may be useful to detect abnormal motion. The best sign of instability is probably the progression of the anterolisthesis on follow-up plain film exams. Computed tomography is the best study to detect early erosive changes in the facets, but these findings are frequently identified in asymptomatic people. Magnetic resonance imaging is useful to detect cartilage erosions or the presence of synovial cysts.

The findings of ankylosing spondylitis are easily assessed on plain films, but spinal fractures in these patients may be difficult to detect on routine radiographs. If there is any question concerning the possibility of a fracture, multiplanar CT or MRI should be obtained quickly because of the potential catastrophic changes that may result from acute instability in these patients. Plain films are also usually adequate in the diagnostic evaluation of the other seronegative spondyloarthropathies, particularly if the patient presents with only back pain.

CONCLUSION

In the evaluation of patients presenting with symptoms related to disorders of the spinal column, plain films are obtained as the first radiologic study. The main value of plain films is to provide general information about the alignment and the condition of the spine; this information can then be supplemented with additional tests if needed. Plain films give an indication of the biomechanical status of the spine and provide information concerning the degree and extent of degenerative processes. Plain films help us to understand the natural history of disorders of the spine and to follow the evolution of a pathologic process. When additional information is needed to solve a specific clinical problem, CT with multiplanar reformations and MRI are both excellent diagnostic tests. The strength of CT resides in its superb demonstration of osseous anatomy, and the strength of MRI is its excellent characterization of soft tissue abnormalities.

One of the greatest challenges in the evaluation of the spine is that myriad diseases may present with similar symptoms (e.g., axial or radicular pain). The algorithm in ordering diagnostic imaging studies is relatively straightforward. Plain films are initially obtained when additional diagnostic information is needed to explain a patient's symptoms. If these do not provide the necessary information, an MRI study is usually the optimal exam to evaluate most clinical conditions. This assumes that the technical quality of the study is excellent and that its interpretation is accurate. This requires a radiologic consultant who is subspecialized in imaging the spine and who thoroughly understands the clinical manifestations of a spectrum of spinal disorders. In cases of spinal trauma and tumors, both CT and MRI are frequently ordered because of the complementary information they provide. Computed tomography-myelography and radionuclide studies have limited application to a few specific clinical situations.

To maximize the amount of information obtained from any imaging study, the clinician should have a working hypothesis as to the potential causes of the spinal dysfunction. The results of the imaging studies become meaningful only when they are integrated with the patient's history, physical exam, and other diagnostic tests. Isolated test results are of little benefit, and they can frequently create more confusion than clarity if there was little indication for obtaining the study. With the complexity of the newer imaging techniques, the radiologist should be an active member of the team of physicians caring for patients with spinal disorders. It is the responsibility of the radiologist to optimize each study to help answer specific clinical questions. With a team approach it should be possible to limit the number of tests ordered and to perform the optimal test to solve different clinical problems.

SUGGESTED READING

1. Atlas SW, ed. *Magnetic resonance imaging of the brain and spine.* New York: Raven Press, 1991.
2. Heitoff KB, Herzog RJ. Computed tomography (CT) and enhanced CT of the spine. In: Frymoyer JW, ed. *The adult spine: principles and practice.* New York: Raven Press, 1991; 335–402.
3. Herzog RJ. Magnetic resonance imaging of the spine. In: Frymoyer JW, ed. *The adult spine: principles and practice.* New York: Raven Press, 1991; 457–510.
4. Modic MT, Masaryk TJ, Ross JS, eds. *Magnetic resonance imaging of the spine.* 2nd ed. Chicago: Year Book Medical Publishers, 1994.
5. Post MJD, ed. *Computed tomography of the spine.* Baltimore: Williams and Wilkins, 1984.

8

Diagnosis and Management of Cervical and Lumbar Disease

Sam W. Wiesel and *Scott D. Boden

*Department of Orthopaedic Surgery, Georgetown University Hospital,
Washington, D.C. 20007, USA; and *Department of Orthopaedic Surgery,
Emory University School of Medicine, Decatur, Georgia 30033, USA*

Key Points

- Symptoms of neck and arm pain may be mechanical, discogenic, or stenotic. One must rule out myelopathy, often associated with gait disturbance.

- Most cervical radiculopathies improve with nonoperative care; most myelopathies do not.

- Symptoms of back and leg pain may be mechanical, discogenic, or stenotic. One must be aware of the findings associated with cauda equina syndrome (i.e., urinary retention, altered perianal sensation, and associated neurologic deficits).

- Acute back pain generally resolves; bed rest, if indicated, should be limited to 3 to 7 days; avoid polypharmacy treatments and narcotics/sedatives.

- Abnormal imaging studies are seen in normal people.

In patients who have undergone multiple operations, diagnostic accuracy affects outcome.

The task of the physician, when confronted with a patient who has neck or low back pain, is to integrate the patient's complaints into an accurate diagnosis and to prescribe appropriate therapy at the proper time. Achieving this goal depends on the accuracy of the physician's thought processes. Although specific information is not available for every aspect of neck or low back pain, there is a large body of data to guide us in handling these patients.

This knowledge can be organized into the format of an algorithm, which can be defined as the solution of a problem (neck or low back pain) in a finite number of steps. It is, in effect, an organized pattern of decision making and thought processes found useful in approaching the universe of cervical and lumbar spine patients. Each diagnostic and treatment decision point is based on established medical practice that can be supported in the current medical literature. It allows the patient to receive the most beneficial diagnostic and therapeutic measures at the optimum times.

This chapter presents algorithms for the cervical spine, the lumbar spine, and the multiply operated patient with low back pain. The use of these algorithms will aid the physician in making efficient and precise use of diagnostic studies, minimizing the use of ineffective surgery, and making therapy available at a reasonable cost to society.

THE CERVICAL
NONOPERATIVE SPINE

The algorithm (see Fig. 1) begins with the universe of patients who are initially evaluated for neck pain with or without arm pain. The differential diagnostic section of the algorithm has also been reformatted in the form of a table (Table 1).

Patients with major trauma including fractures are not included. After an initial medical history and physical examination and with the assumption that the patient's symptoms are originating from the cervical spine, the first major decision is to rule in or out the presence of a cervical myelopathy.

The character and severity of the myelopathy depends on the size, location, and duration of the lesion. Ventrolateral lesions encroach on the nerve roots and lateral aspects of the spinal cord, producing all of the manifestations accompanying nerve root compression. The chief radicular signs are weakness and loss of tone and volume of the muscles of the upper extremity, and the pressure on the spinal cord may produce pyramidal tract signs and spasticity in the lower extremities.

Midline lesions intrude on the central aspect of the anterior portion of the spinal cord. They produce no signs of nerve root compression. Both lower extremities are primarily involved, and the most common problem relates initially to gait disturbances. As the disease progresses, bowel and bladder control may be affected.

Once a diagnosis of a cervical myelopathy is made, surgical intervention should be considered quickly. The best results are attained in patients with one or two motor units involved and with a myelopathy of a relatively short duration. The longer pressure is applied to the neural elements, the poorer the results. A cervical MRI or CT-myelogram, if necessary, should be obtained in these patients to define the neural compression precisely, and an adequate surgical decompression should be performed as soon as possible to achieve the best results.

After a cervical myelopathy has been ruled out, the remaining patients, who

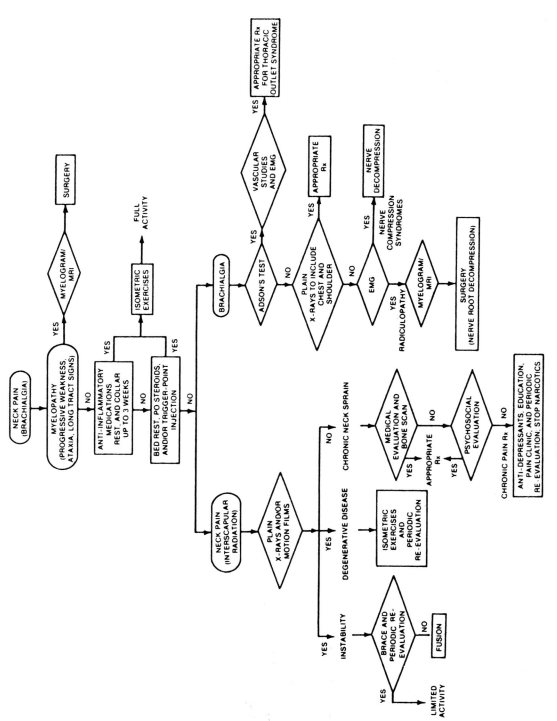

FIG. 1. Cervical spine algorithm.

TABLE 1. *The differential diagnosis of neck pain*

Evaluation	Neck strain	HNP	Instability	Degenerative disc disease	Myelopathy	Tumor	Spondyloarthropathy	Metabolic	Infection
Predominant pain	Neck	Arm	Neck	Neck	Neck	Neck	Neck	Neck	Neck
Constitutional symptoms						+	+	+/−	+
Compression test		+							
Neurologic exam		+			+				
Plain x-rays			+/−	+	+/−	+/−	+	+	+/−
Lateral motion x-rays			+						
CT	+		+	+/−	+			+	
Myelogram		+			+				
MRI		+	+		+	+		+	+
Bone scan						+	+	+/−	+
ESR							+		+
Ca/P/Alk phos								+	

HNP, herniated nucleus pulposus; CT, computed tomography; ESR, erythrocyte sedimentation rate; Ca, calcium; P, phosphorous; Alk phos, alkaline phosphatase.

constitute an overwhelming majority, should be started on a course of conservative management. At this stage of the patient's course, a specific diagnosis, whether it be a herniated disc or neck strain, is not important because the entire group is treated in the same fashion.

Conservative Treatment

The primary mode of therapy in both acute and chronic cervical spine disease is immobilization. In acute neck injuries immobilization allows healing of torn and attenuated soft tissues, whereas in chronic conditions immobilization is aimed at reduction of inflammation in the supporting soft tissues and nerve roots of the cervical spine. Immobilization is best achieved by the use of a soft collar. It must be properly fitted and comfortable for the patient. Initially the collar is worn 24 hr a day. The patient must understand that during sleep the neck is totally unprotected from awkward positions and movement and that the collar is most important.

The other mainstay of the initial treatment is drug therapy. It is directed at reducing inflammation—especially in the soft tissues. A variety of anti-inflammatory medications are available; however, no one drug has proven to be significantly better than all of the others. Salicylates have proven to be as effective and safe as the rest and are least expensive. The dosage must be adequate to achieve a therapeutic blood level. The efficacy of this treatment regimen is predicated on the patient's ability to understand the disease process and the role of each therapeutic modality. The vast majority of patients will respond to this approach during the first 10 days, but a certain percentage will not.

At this juncture a local injection into the area of maximum tenderness may be considered. Localized tender areas in the paravertebral musculature and trapezii, referred to as *trigger points,* will be found in many individuals. Marked relief of symptoms often is achieved dramatically by infiltration of these trigger points with a combination of lidocaine (Xylocaine) and 1 ml of a steroid preparation. The object of the injection is to decrease the inflammation in a specific anatomic area. The more localized the trigger point, the more effective this form of therapy.

The patient should, when possible, be treated conservatively for up to 6 wk. The majority of cervical spine patients will get better and should be encouraged to increase their activities gradually. The goal is a return to their normal lifestyles. The exercise should be directed at strengthening the paravertebral musculature, not at increasing the range of motion.

This portion of the algorithm is reversible. Should regression occur—with exacerbation of symptoms—the physician can resort to more stringent conservative measures, which may include additional bed rest and stronger anti-inflammatory medication. The majority of patients with neck pain will respond to therapy and return to a normal life pattern within 2 mo of the beginning of their problem. If the initial conservative treatment regimen fails, symptomatic patients are divided into two groups. The first comprises people with neck pain as a predominant complaint, with or without interscapular radiation. The second group is made up of those who complain primarily of arm pain (brachialgia).

Patients with Neck Pain Predominant

After 6 wk of conservative therapy with no symptomatic relief, plain radiographs with lateral flexion-extension films are carefully examined for abnormalities. One group of patients will have objective evidence of instability. In the lower cervical spine (C3-7), hypermobility is identified by horizontal translation of one vertebra on another of more than 3.5 mm or by an angular difference of adjacent vertebrae of more than 11°. The majority of patients with hypermobility will respond well to further nonoperative measures, including a thorough explanation of the problem and some type of bracing. In some cases, these measures will fail and a surgical fusion of the involved spinal segments will be necessary.

Another group of patients complaining mainly of neck pain will have evidence of degenerative disease on their plain radiographs. The radiographic signs include loss of height of the intervertebral disc space, osteophyte formation, secondary encroachment of the intervertebral foramina, and osteoarthritic changes in the apophyseal joint. The difficulty is not in identifying these abnormalities on the radiograph but in determining their significance.

Degeneration in the cervical spine can be a normal part of the aging process. In a study of matched pairs of asymptomatic and symptomatic patients, it was concluded that a large number of asymptomatic patients show radiographic evidence of advanced degenerative disease. The most significant radiographic finding relevant to symptoms was found to be narrowing of the intervertebral disc space, particularly between C5-6 and C6-7. There was no difference between the two groups as far as changes at the apophyseal joints, intervertebral foramina, or posterior articular processes.

These patients should be treated symptomatically with anti-inflammatory medications, support, and trigger point injections as required. In the quiescent stages they should be placed on isometric exercises. Finally, they should be re-examined periodically because some will develop significant pressure on the neurologic elements (myelopathy) with the passage of time.

The majority of patients with neck pain will have normal radiographs. The diagnosis often given to this group is neck strain, which remains ill defined. At this point, with no objective findings, other abnormalities must be considered. These patients should undergo a bone scan and medical evaluation. The bone scan can be an excellent tool, often identifying early spinal tumors or infections not seen on routine radiographic examinations. A thorough medical search also may reveal problems missed in the early stages of neck pain evaluation. If these diagnostic studies are positive, the patient is treated appropriately.

If the above work-up is negative, the patient should have a thorough psychosocial evaluation. This is predicated on the belief that patients' disability is related not only to pathologic anatomy but also to their perception of pain and stability in relationship to the sociologic environment. Drug habituation, alcoholism, depression, and other psychiatric problems frequently are seen in association with neck pain. If the evaluation reveals this type of problem, proper nonoperative measures are instituted to overcome the disability.

Should the psychosocial evaluation prove normal, the patient is considered to have chronic neck pain. One must be aware that other outside factors such as compensation and/or litigation can influence a patient's perception of subjective pain. Patients with chronic neck pain need encouragement, patience, and education from their physicians. They need to be detoxified from narcotic drugs and placed on an exercise regimen. Many will respond to antidepressant drugs such as amitriptyline. All of these patients need periodic reevaluation to avoid missing any new or underlying pathologic condition.

Patients with Arm Pain Predominant (Brachialgia)

Patients who have pain radiating into their arm may be experiencing symptoms secondary to mechanical pressure and inflammation of the involved nerve roots. This mechanical pressure may arise from a ruptured disc or from bone secondary to degenerative changes. Other pathologic causes of arm pain should be carefully considered. Extrinsic pressure on the vascular structures or on the peripheral nerves is the most likely imitator of brachialgia. Abnormality in the chest and shoulder also should be ruled out.

A careful physical examination should be conducted. If there is any question about the cause of the findings, appropriate radiographs, an MRI/CT, and neurodiagnostic studies such as an electromyogram (EMG) should be obtained. If any of these is indicative of peripheral pressure on the nerves or other pathologic conditions (tumor), the appropriate therapy should be instituted.

If the findings are consistent with mechanical pressure on the cervical elements from either a herniated nucleus pulposus (HNP), an osteophyte, or a combination of the two, the patient is considered to have brachialgia. These patients, for whom nonoperative treatment has failed, should be considered for surgical decompression at this juncture.

It has been documented repeatedly that, for surgery to be effective, unequivocal evidence of nerve root compression must be found at surgery. One must have firm confirmation of mechanical root compression from the neurologic examination and a confirming study before proceeding with any surgery. The indications for surgery are the subjective complaint of arm pain and a neurologic deficit or positive MRI. If the patient does not have these, there is inadequate clinical evidence of root compression to proceed with surgery, regardless of the investigative findings. For individuals who have met these criteria for cervical decompression, the results will usually be satisfactory: 95% of them can expect good or excellent results.

THE LUMBAR SPINE

As with patients with neck pain, the task of the physician when confronted with the patient with low back pain is to integrate the patient's complaints into an accurate diagnosis and to prescribe appropriate therapy. This problem (universe of low back pain patients) has been formatted into an algorithm (see Fig. 2), the aim of which is to select the correct diagnostic category and proper treatment avenues for each patient with low back pain. A specific patient may fall outside the limits of the algorithm and require a different approach, and the physician must constantly be on the alert for exceptions. The algorithm is presented in table form in Table 2.

The information necessary to use the algorithm is initially obtained through the history and physical examination. The key points in the history are differentiating back pain that is mechanical in nature from nonmechanical pain that is present at rest, detecting changes in bowel or bladder function, and defining the precise location and quality of the pain. The physical examination must be oriented toward ruling out other medical causes of low back pain, assessing neurologic function, and evaluating for the presence of tension signs.

Following the low back pain algorithm, the first major decision is to make a ruling on the presence or absence of cauda equina compression (CEC) syndrome. Mechanical compression of the cauda equina, with truly progressive motor weakness, is one of the few surgical emergencies in lumbar spine patients. This compression usually is due to pressure on the caudal sac, through which pass the nerves to the lower extremities, bowel, and bladder. The signs and symptoms are a complex mixture of those of low back pain, which can be subtle bilateral motor weakness of the lower extremities, bilateral sciatica, saddle anesthesia, and even

frank paraplegia with bowel and bladder incontinence. Cauda equina compression can be caused by either bone or soft tissue damage, the latter generally in the form of a ruptured or herniated disc in the midline. These patients should undergo an immediate definitive diagnostic test and, if it is positive, emergency surgical decompression.

Historically, the myelogram was the study used in this setting; however, the development of MRI has facilitated the noninvasive diagnosis of CEC. The principal reason for prompt surgical intervention is to arrest the progression of neurologic loss; the chance of actual return of lost neurologic function after surgery is small. Although the incidence of CEC in the entire back pain population is very low, it is one of the only entities that requires immediate operative intervention; if its diagnosis is missed, the consequences can be devastating.

The remaining patients make up the overwhelming majority. They should be started on a course of conservative (nonoperative) therapy regardless of the diagnosis. At this stage the specific diagnosis, whether a herniated disc or back pain, cause unknown, is not important to the therapy because the entire population is treated the same way. A few of these patients will eventually need an invasive procedure (surgery), but at this point there is no way to predict which individuals will respond to conservative therapy and which will not.

Conservative Nonoperative Treatment

The vast majority in this initial group have nonradiating low back pain, termed

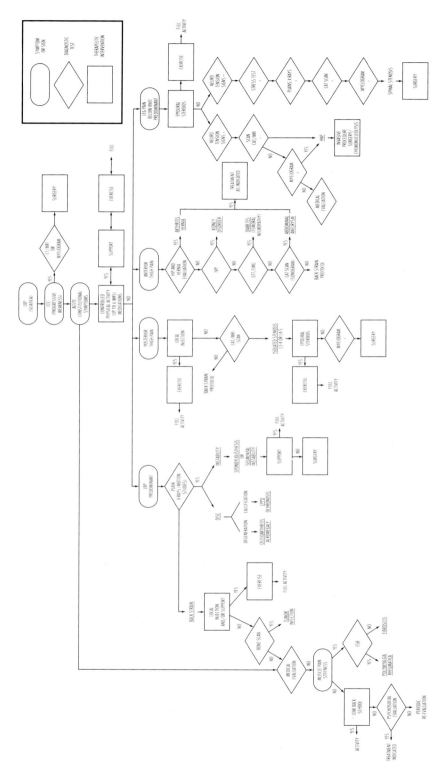

FIG. 2. Low back pain algorithm.

TABLE 2. *The differential diagnosis of low back pain*

Evaluation	Back strain	HNP	Spinal stenosis	Spondylolisthesis/instability	Spondyloarthropathy	Infection	Tumor	Metabolic	Hematologic	Visceral
Predominant pain	Back	Leg (below knee)	Back/leg	Back/leg	Back	Back	Back	Back	Back	Back (buttock/thigh)
Constitutional symptoms					+	+	+/−	+	+	+
Tension sign		+		+/−						
Neurologic exam		+/−	+/− after stress				+/−			
Plain x-rays			+	+	+	+/−	+/−	+	+	
Lateral motion x-rays				+						
CT/MRI		+	+				+			+
Myelogram		+	+							
Bone scan					+	+	+	+	+	
ESR					+	+	+	+	+	+
Serum chemistries							+	+	+	+

MRI, magnetic resonance imaging.

lumbago or *back strain.* The cause of lumbago is not clear. There are several possibilities, including ligamentous or muscular injuries, continuous mechanical stress from poor posture, facet joint irritation, or a small tear in the annulus fibrosis. Patients usually complain of pain in the low back, often localized to a single area. On physical examination they demonstrate a decreased range of lumbar spine motion, tenderness to palpation over the involved area, and paraspinal muscle spasm. Their radiographic examinations usually are normal, but, if therapy is not successful, films should be obtained to rule out other possible etiologic factors. Two exceptions to this rule are patients younger than 20 yr and patients over age 50; radiographs are important early in the diagnostic process because these patients may be more likely to have a diagnosis other than nonspecific back pain (i.e., tumor or infection). Other situations warranting radiography sooner rather than later include a history of serious trauma, known cancer, unexplained weight loss, fever, or other constitutional symptoms.

The early stage of the treatment of low back pain (with or without leg pain) is a waiting game. The passage of time, the use of anti-inflammatory medication, and controlled physical activity are the modalities proven safest and most effective. The vast majority of these patients will respond to this approach within the first 10 days, although a small percentage will not. In today's society, with its emphasis on quick solutions and "high technology," many patients are pushed too rapidly toward more complex (i.e., invasive) management. This "quick fix" approach has no

place in the treatment of low back pain. The physician should treat the patient conservatively and wait up to at least 6 wk for a response. As already stated, most of these patients will improve within 10 days—a few will take longer.

Once the patients have achieved approximately 80% relief, they should be mobilized with the help of a lightweight, flexible corset. After they are more comfortable and have increased their activity level, they should begin a program of isometric lumbar exercises and return to their normal lifestyles. This section of the protocol is a two-way street: should regression occur with exacerbation of symptoms, the physician can resort to more stringent conservative measures. The patient may require further bed rest. Most acute low back pain patients will proceed along this pathway, returning to their normal life patterns within 2 mo of the onset of symptoms. In most cases bed rest should not exceed 3 to 7 days.

If the initial conservative treatment regimen fails and 6 wk have passed, symptomatic patients are sorted into four groups. The first group is composed of people with low back pain predominating. The second group complains mainly of leg pain, defined as pain radiating below the knee and commonly referred to as *sciatica.* The third group has posterior thigh pain. The fourth group has anterior thigh pain. Each group follows a separate diagnostic and treatment pathway.

Patients with Predominating Low Back Pain

Those patients who continue to complain predominantly of low back pain at

6 wk should have plain radiographs carefully examined for abnormalities. Spondylolysis with or without spondylolisthesis is the most common structural abnormality to cause significant low back pain. Approximately 5% of the population has this defect, thought to be caused by a combination of genetics and environmental stress. In spite of this defect, most of these people are able to perform their activities of daily living with little or no discomfort. When symptoms are present, these patients usually will respond to nonoperative measures, including a thorough explanation of the problem, a back support, and exercises. In a small percentage of such cases, conservative treatment fails and a fusion of the involved spinal segments becomes necessary. This is one of the few times primary fusion of the lumbar spine is indicated, and it must be stressed that it is a relatively infrequent occurrence.

The vast majority of patients with pain predominantly in the low back will have normal plain radiographs. The diagnosis at this point is back strain. Before there is any additional work-up, a local injection of steroids and lidocaine may be tried at the point of maximum tenderness. This can be quite successful, and, if there is a good response, the patient is begun on exercises with gradual resumption of normal activity. In some instances, if there are no objective findings, such a trigger point injection can be considered as early as the third week after onset of symptoms

Should the patient not respond to a local injection, other abnormalities must be seriously considered. A bone scan and MRI, along with a general medical evaluation, should be obtained.

The bone scan is an excellent tool, often identifying early bone tumors or infections not visible on routine radiographic examinations. It is particularly important to obtain this study in the patient with nonmechanical back pain. If the pain is constant, unremitting, and unrelieved by postural adjustments, more often than not the correct diagnosis will be one of an occult neoplasm or metabolic disorder not readily apparent from other testing. The MRI is very useful as a screening tool to rule out intraspinal abnormality, such as a neurofibroma.

Approximately 3% of patients with apparent low back pain who present at orthopaedic clinics have pain attributable to extraspinal causes. A thorough medical search also frequently reveals problems missed earlier, such as a posterior penetrating ulcer, pancreatitis, renal disease, or an abdominal aneurysm. If these diagnostic studies are positive, the patient should be transferred into a nonorthopaedic treatment service and would no longer fit into the therapeutic algorithm.

Those patients who have no abnormality on their bone scans and do not show other medical disease as a cause for their back pain are then referred for another type of therapy—the low back school. It is believed that many of these patients are suffering from discogenic pain or facet joint pain syndrome. The low back school concept has as its basis the belief that patients with low back pain, given proper education and understanding of their disease, often can return to a productive and functional life. Ergonomics, the proper and efficient use of the spine in work and recreation, is stressed. Back school need not be an expensive proposition. It can be a one-time classroom session with a review of back problems and a demonstration of exercise with patient participation. This type of educational process has proved very effective. It is most important, however, that the patient be thoroughly screened before being referred to this type of program. One does not want to be in the position of treating a metastatic tumor in a classroom.

If low back school is not successful, the patient should undergo a thorough psychosocial evaluation in an attempt to explain the failure of the previous treatments. This is predicated on the knowledge that a patient's ability is related not only to the pathologic anatomy but also to the patient's perception of pain and stability in relation to the social environment. It is quite common to see a stable patient with a frank herniated disc continue working—regarding the disability as only a minor problem—while a hysterical patients takes to bed at the slightest twinge of low back discomfort.

Drug habituation, depression, alcoholism, and other psychiatric problems are seen frequently in association with back pain. If the evaluation suggests any of these problems, proper measures should be instituted to overcome the disability. There are a surprising number of ambulatory patients addicted to commonly prescribed medications using complaints of back pain as an excuse to obtain these drugs. Oxycodone and diazepam, alone or in combination, are the two most popular offenders. Oxy-

codone is truly addictive; diazepam is both habituating and depressing. Since the complaint of low back pain may be a common manifestation of depression, it is counterproductive to treat such patients with diazepam.

Approximately 2% of patients who initially present with low back pain will fail treatment and elude any diagnosis. There will be no evidence of any structural problem in the back or criteria for underlying medical disease or psychiatric disorder. This is a very difficult group to manage. The author's strategy has been to discontinue narcotics, reassure the patient, and periodically re-evaluate. Over time, one third of these patients will be found to have an underlying medical disease; thus, one cannot abandon this group and discontinue treatment. For the remainder, as much physical activity as possible should be encouraged.

Patients with Sciatica

The next group of patients consists of those with sciatica, which is pain radiating below the knees. These patients usually experience their symptoms secondary to mechanical pressure and inflammation of the nerve roots that originate in the back and extend down the leg. The mechanical pressure can be due to soft tissue (herniated disc), bone, or a combination of the two.

At this point in the algorithm, the patient has had up to 6 wk of controlled physical activity and medication but still has persistent leg pain. The next therapeutic step is an epidural steroid injection, which is performed on an outpatient basis. An epidural injection is worth trying; the chance of success is 40% and morbidity is low, particularly compared with the next treatment step—surgery. The maximum benefit from a single injection is often achieved by 2 wk. The injection may have to be repeated once or twice, and 4 to 6 wk should pass before its success or failure is judged. Generally no more than three injections in one year are recommended.

If epidural steroids are effective in alleviating the patient's leg pain or sciatica, he or she is begun on a program of back exercises and encouraged to return promptly to as normal a lifestyle as possible. Should the epidural steroids prove ineffective and 3 months have passed since the initial injury without relief of pain, some type of invasive treatment should be considered. The patient group is then divided into those with probable herniated discs and those with symptoms secondary to spinal stenosis.

The physician must now carefully re-evaluate the patient for a neurologic deficit and for positive tension sign(s) [i.e., the straight leg raise test (SLRT)]. For those who have either a neurologic deficit or positive tension signs along with continued leg pain, a CT scan or MRI should be obtained. If either the CT scan or the MRI is clearly positive and correlates with the clinical findings, myelography no longer need be performed, since it is invasive. If there is any question about the findings, one should proceed with the other noninvasive study not yet done (CT or MRI) or a metrizamide myelogram.

As in the cervical spine, there is repeated documentation that, for surgery to be effective in the treatment of a her-niated disc, the surgeon must find unequivocal operative evidence of nerve root compression. Accordingly, nerve root compression must be firmly substantiated preoperatively, not only by neurologic examination but also by radiographic data. There is no place for "exploratory" spine surgery. Many asymptomatic patients have been found to have abnormal myelograms, EMGs, CT scans, and MR images. If the patient has neither a neurologic deficit nor a positive SLRT, regardless of radiographic findings, there is not enough evidence of root compression to proceed with surgery. The patients without objective findings are the ones who have poor results and have given back surgery a bad name.

If there are no objective findings, the physician should avoid surgery and proceed to the psychosocial evaluation. Exceptions should be few and far between. When sympathy for the patient's complaints outweighs the objective evaluation, surgery is fraught with difficulties. For those patients who meet these specific criteria for lumbar laminectomy, results will be satisfactory: 95% of them can expect a good to excellent result.

The second group of patients whose symptoms are based on mechanical pressure on the neural elements are those with spinal stenosis. The diagnosis of spinal stenosis usually can be made from the plain radiographs, which will demonstrate facet degeneration, disc degeneration, and decreased interpedicular and sagittal canal diameters. A CT scan and/or MRI can confirm the diagnosis. If symptoms are severe and there is radiographic evidence of spinal stenosis, surgery is appropriate. Age alone is not a deterrent to surgery; many elderly people who are in good health except for a narrow spinal canal will benefit greatly from adequate decompression of the lumbar spine.

Patients with Anterior Thigh Pain

A small percentage of patients will have pain that radiates from the back into the anterior thighs. This usually is relieved by rest and anti-inflammatory medication. If the discomfort persists after 6 wk of treatment, a work-up should be initiated to search for underlying pathologic conditions. Several entities must be considered.

A hip problem or hernia can be ruled out with a thorough physical examination. If the hip examination is positive, radiographs should be obtained. An intravenous pyelogram is useful to evaluate the urinary tract because kidney stones often may present as anterior thigh pain. Peripheral neuropathy, most commonly secondary to diabetes, also can present initially with anterior thigh pain; a glucose tolerance test as well as an EMG will reveal the underlying problem. Finally, a retroperitoneal tumor can cause symptoms by mechanically pressing on the nerves that innervate the anterior thighs. A CT scan or MR image of the retroperitoneal area will eliminate or confirm this possibility. Remember, lateral disc herniation in the upper lumbar spine must be ruled out by MRI or CT.

If any of the entities reviewed above is diagnosed, the patient is treated accordingly. If no physical cause can be found for the anterior thigh pain, the patient is treated for recalcitrant back strain by the method already outlined.

Patients with Posterior Thigh Pain

This final group of patients will complain of back pain with radiation into the buttocks and posterior thighs. Most of them will be relieved of their symptoms with 6 wk of conservative therapy. However, if their pain persists after the initial treatment period, they can be considered to have back strain and be given a trigger point injection of steroids and lidocaine in the area of maximum tenderness. If the injection is unsuccessful, it is necessary to distinguish between referred and radicular pain.

Referred pain is pain in the mesodermal tissues of the same embryologic origin. The muscles, tendons, and ligaments of the buttocks and posterior thighs have the same embryologic origin as those of the low back. When the low back is injured, pain may be referred to the posterior thighs, where it is perceived by the patient. Referred pain from irritated soft tissues cannot be cured with a surgical procedure.

Radicular pain is caused by compression of an inflamed nerve root along the anatomic course of the nerve. A herniated disc or spinal stenosis in the high lumbar area can cause radiation of pain into the posterior thigh. Magnetic resonance imaging or CT and an EMG may be used in this situation to differentiate radicular etiology from referred pain or a peripheral nerve lesion. If the studies are within normal limits, the patient is considered to have nonradicular back pain (some refer to this as *back strain*) and is treated according to the algorithm. If a radicular abnormality is found, the patient is diagnosed as having mechanical compression of the neural elements from either a herniated disc or spinal stenosis. Epidural steroids should be tried first; if these do not provide adequate relief, surgery should be contemplated.

This group of patients with unexplained posterior thigh pain is very difficult to treat. The biggest mistake made is the performance of surgery on patients thought to have radicular pain who actually have referred pain. Again, referred pain in this setting is not responsive to surgery.

In most instances the treatment of low back pain is no longer a mystery. The algorithm described here presents a series of easy-to-follow and clearly defined decision-making processes. Use of this algorithm provides you with helpful diagnostic and therapeutic measures at specific time intervals. It neither denies patients helpful surgery, when indicated, nor subjects them to procedures that are useless technical exercises.

THE MULTIPLY OPERATED LUMBAR SPINE

The evaluation and treatment of the patient with previous back surgery is a challenging problem. It is estimated that 300,000 new laminectomies are performed each year in the United States alone and that 15% of these patients will continue to have significant pain. The inherent complexity of these cases necessitates a specific method of problem solving that is precise and unambiguous.

The best possible solution for preventing continued symptoms after spine surgery is to prevent inappropriate surgery before it occurs. If proper surgical indications for the initial procedure were strictly followed, this would probably prevent recurrent symptoms in a large number of patients. The idea of exploring the low back when the necessary objective criteria are not met is no longer acceptable. In fact, even when there are objective findings but the patient is psychologically unstable or there are compensation/litigation factors, the outcome of back surgery is questionable and it should be undertaken only after careful deliberation. Thus, the initial decision to operate is the most important one. Once the situation of pain after the operation has arisen, the potential for a solution is limited at best.

In the evaluation of recurrent symptoms after surgery, the problem confronting the physician is to distinguish the patient with a mechanical lesion from the patient whose symptoms are secondary to nonmechanical problems. The types of mechanical lesions include recurrent herniated discs, spinal instability, and spinal stenosis. These three entities produce symptoms by causing direct pressure on the neural elements and in some cases are amenable to further surgical intervention. The nonmechanical entities consist of scar tissue (either arachnoiditis or epidural fibrosis), psychosocial instability, or systemic medical disease. These nonmechanical problems will not be helped by any type of additional spine surgery.

The keystone for successful treatment is to obtain an accurate diagnosis. Although a seemingly obvious need, this essential step is often not taken. Consequently, the rehabilitation of this patient

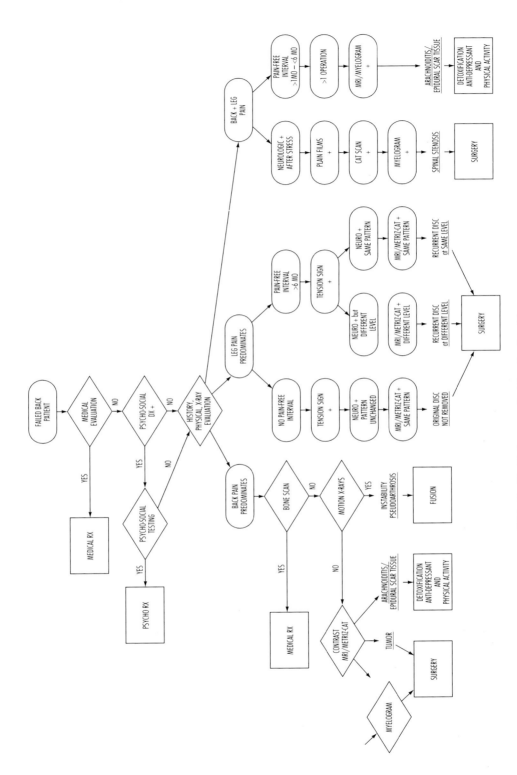

FIG. 3. Multiply operated back algorithm.

TABLE 3. *The differential diagnosis of the multiply operated back*

History-physical radiographs	Original disc not removed	Recurrent disc at same level	Recurrent disc at different level	Spinal instability	Spinal stenosis	Arachnoiditis	Epidural scar tissue	Discitis
Number of previous operations						>1		>1
Pain-free interval	None	>6 mo	>6 mo			>1 mo, but <6 mo	>1 mo gradual onset	
Predominant pain	Leg pain	Leg pain	Leg pain	Back pain	Back and leg pain	Back and leg pain	Back and or leg pain	Back pain
Tension sign	+	+	+			May be positive	May be positive	
Neurologic exam	+ same pattern	+ same pattern	+ different level		+ after stress			
Plain x-rays	+ if wrong level				+			+/–
Lateral motion x-rays				+				
Metrizamide myelogram	+ but unchanged	+ same level	+ different level		+	+	+	
CAT scan	+	+	+		+	+	+ (IV contrast)	+ (IV contrast)
MRI	+	+	+		+	+	+ (gadolinium contrast)	+

group has been fraught with difficulty. The algorithm is presented in Fig. 3 and the differential diagnosis is formatted in Table 3.

Evaluation

When a multiply operated back patient first arrives for evaluation, it is important to obtain all of the vital information in an organized manner. Obtaining the radiographs and past history to review before the patient is actually seen is most helpful. The use of a standardized form will lessen the chance of missing significant details. These steps are important because these patients are extremely difficult to evaluate.

The evaluation of the multiply operated back patient must begin with the history, which can be extremely complicated. Many patients want to relate their entire story to the evaluating physician, and it is probably best to let them do so. However, after the patient finishes this story, three specific historical points must be elucidated so that the proper decision-making process can be initiated. The first is the number of previous lumbar spine operations the patient has undergone. It has been shown in several studies that, with every subsequent operation, regardless of the diagnosis, the percentage of good results diminishes. Statistically, the second operation has a 50% chance of success, and beyond two operations patients are more likely to be made worse than better.

The next important historical point is the length of the pain-free interval after the patient's previous operation. If the patient awakes from surgery with pain still present, it is likely that the nerve root may not have been properly decompressed or that the wrong level was explored. If the pain-free interval was at least 6 mo, the patient's recurrent pain may be on the basis of another herniation of disc material at the same or a different level. If the pain-free interval was between 1 and 6 mo and recurrent symptoms had a gradual onset, the diagnosis may be some type of scar tissue, either arachnoiditis or epidural fibrosis.

Finally, the patient's pain pattern must be evaluated. If the pain predominates, a herniated disc or spinal stenosis is most likely, although scar tissue is also a possibility. If back pain is the major component, instability, tumor, infection, and scar tissue are the major considerations. If both back pain and leg pain are present, spinal stenosis and scar tissue are the likely possibilities.

Physical examination is the next major step in the evaluation of the multiply operated back patient. The neurologic findings and existence of a tension sign, such as the sitting straight-leg-raising test, must be noted. It is helpful to have the results of a dependable previous examination so a comparison between the preoperative and postoperative states can be made. If the neurologic picture is unchanged from before the previous surgery and the tension sign is negative, mechanical pressure is unlikely. If, however, a new neurologic deficit has occurred since the last surgery or the tension sign is positive, pressure on the neural elements is possible. One must realize that epidural or perineural fibrosis can cause a positive tension sign; the tension sign is not pathognomonic for a mechanical lesion in the setting of patients with previous spine surgery.

Roentgenographic studies are the last major part of the patient's work-up. It is most helpful to have studies that were performed before the previous surgical procedure for comparison of the preoperative and postoperative situation. Often careful analysis may reveal that the initial operation was not indicated.

The plain radiograph must be evaluated for the extent and level of the previous laminectomies and for any evidence of spinal stenosis. It should not be taken for granted that the correct level was decompressed; the laminectomy level on the plain radiograph must correspond to the level on the preoperative radiographic studies, to the level described in the operative report, and to the neurologic findings demonstrated by the patient. The standing (weight-bearing) lateral-flexion-extension radiographs must be assessed for any evidence of abnormal motion; this will be discussed in further detail under lumbar instability in the differential diagnosis section.

Metrizamide myelography in the multiply operated back patient with chronic pain can be of some value. Although this test can identify extradural compressions, myelography cannot distinguish between disc material and epidural scar tissue. The major information obtained from myelography is used for confirming arachnoiditis when the diagnosis is otherwise uncertain. Computed tomography (CT) scanning following metrizamide injection in the subarachnoid space is also a sensitive test for demonstrating the changes of arachnoiditis.

Magnetic resonance imaging (MRI) with gadolinium is also a very useful tool in these patients to try to distinguish a recurrent disc herniation from epidural scar tissue. A herniated disc is avascular and will not enhance (light up) immediately after the injection of gadolinium; scar tissue, on the other hand, is vascular and will enhance on the scan. The diagnostic accuracy at this time has been shown to approach 100% in a surgically and histologically confirmed series. However in another study gadolinium MR of the asymptomatic postoperative lumbar spine during the first six months revealed pathologic changes including persistent herniated disc material in 40% despite the complete relief of symptoms. Thus MR scans during the initial six months postoperative period must be interpreted with extreme caution. Finally, the MRI is also a very good screening tool for other types of processes that can cause back pain and may be the etiology for the continued symptoms after previous low back surgery. These include metabolic abnormalities, infections, and tumors of the spine.

The Multiply Operated Low Back Algorithm

The primary goal in the evaluation of the multiply operated back patient is to correctly identify the specific diagnosis. Although a seemingly obvious step, this is many times not done. The most common lesions accounting for failed back surgery syndrome include recurrent or persistent disc herniation (12% to 16%), lateral (58%) or central (7% to 14%) stenosis, arachnoiditis (6% to 16%), epidural fibrosis (6% to 8%), and instability (<5%).

The first step in the algorithm is to determine if the patient's complaint is based on a nonorthopaedic cause, such as pancreatitis, diabetes, or an abdominal aneurysm. Thus, a thorough general medical examination should be routinely obtained. If this examination reveals a systemic problem, it should be treated appropriately. In addition, the patient's psychosocial makeup should also be evaluated and specific items, such as alcoholism, drug dependence, depression, or compensation/litigation should be sought. It has been clearly demonstrated that persons with profound emotional disturbances and those involved with litigation do not derive any significant benefit from additional surgery. Even if a specific orthopaedic diagnosis is made, psychosocial problems should be addressed first. In many cases, once a patient's underlying psychosocial problem has been treated successfully, the somatic back complaints and disability will disappear.

Once the patients with medical and psychosocial problems are identified and separated, the physician is left with a group of people who have back or leg pain. The goal is then to separate those patients with specific mechanical problems from those whose symptoms are secondary to some form of scar tissue or inflammation. The former may benefit from additional surgery; the latter will not. It must be stressed that the incidence of surgically correctable problems is quite low.

The Herniated Intervertebral Disc

Three possibilities exist if the patient's pain is caused by a herniated disc. First, the disc that caused the original symptoms may not have been satisfactorily removed. This can happen if the wrong level was decompressed, the laminectomy performed was not adequate to free the neural elements, or a fragment of disc material was left behind. Such patients will continue to have pain because of mechanical pressure and irritation of the same nerve root that caused the original symptoms. They will complain predominantly of leg pain, and their neurologic findings, tension signs, and radiographic patterns will remain unchanged from the preoperative state. The distinguishing feature is that they will report no pain-free intervals; they will have awakened from the operation complaining of the same preoperative pain. Patients in this group will be helped by a technically correctly performed discectomy.

A second possibility is that there is a recurrent herniated intervertebral disc at the previously decompressed level. These patients complain of sciatica and have unchanged neurologic findings, tension signs, and radiographic studies. The distinguishing characteristic here is that their pain-free interval is usually >6 months. Another operative procedure is indicated in patients with this situation, provided that the contrast-enhanced CT or MRI can demonstrate herniated disc material as the cause of the pressure on the neural elements rather than just scar tissue.

Finally, a herniated disc may occur at a completely different level. Such patients generally will have a pain-free interval >6 months and suffer the sudden onset of recurrent pain. Sciatica will predominate and tension signs are positive. However, a neurologic deficit, if present, and the radiographic findings will occur at a different level from the original studies. A repeat operation for these patients will be beneficial.

Lumbar Instability

Lumbar instability or hypermobility is another condition causing pain on a mechanical basis in the multiply operated back patient. Instability or hypermobility is the abnormal or excessive movement of one vertebra on another causing pain. The etiology may be the patient's intrinsic back disease, such as spondylolisthesis or an excessively wide bilateral laminectomy. Pseudarthrosis resulting from a failed spine fusion is included in this category because its pain would be caused by the instability created by the failed fusion.

Patients with instability will complain predominantly of back pain and their physical examination may be negative. Sometimes, the key to diagnosis of these patients is the weight-bearing, lateral-flexion-extension radiograph; however, it is often difficult to define precisely the anatomic origin of back pain in the presence of radiographic instability. Relative flexion/sagittal plane translation of >12% of the anteroposterior diameter of the ver-

tebral body or relative flexion/sagittal plane rotation of >11° between segments are the most commonly cited guidelines for instability of the lumbar spine. At the lumbosacral junction the criteria are slightly different: relative translation of >25% or rotation of >19% is significant. These criteria are based on maximum displacements on a single flexion or extension view; however, dynamic measurements of relative translation and rotation from flexion or extension may prove to be a more reliable indication of true instability.

Unfortunately, there is little information on why some patients with segmental instability develop back pain, yet others do not. If there is radiographic evidence of instability in symptomatic patients, spinal fusion (or repair of the pseudarthrosis) may be considered. Additional confirmatory evidence to determine the precise level of origin of the patient's symptoms may be gathered from such studies as facet injections and discography; however, these tests have a substantial rate of false-positive results. It should also be pointed out that many patients who have known pseudarthrosis are asymptomatic, and one should be extremely careful.

Spinal Stenosis

Spinal stenosis in the multiply operated back patient can mechanically produce back or leg pain or both. The cause may be secondary to progression of the patient's inherent degenerative spine disease, a previous inadequate decompression, or overgrowth of a previous posterior fusion. The physical examination is usually inconclusive, although a neurologic deficit may occur after exercise with reproduction of the patient's symptoms; this phenomenon is termed a *positive stress test.*

The plain radiographs can be suggestive and may display facet degeneration, decreased interpedicular distance, decreased sagittal canal diameter, and disc degeneration. A CT scan will demonstrate bony encroachment on the neural elements; this is especially helpful in evaluating the lateral recesses and neural foramina. A metrizamide myelogram or MRI will show compression of the dural sac at the involved levels. It should be appreciated that spinal stenosis and scar tissue can coexist. Good results can be expected from surgery in at least 70% of properly selected cases, whereas surgery in those with previous laminectomy and spinal fusion is less successful. If definite evidence of bony compression is present, a laminectomy is indicated; however, if substantial scar tissue is present the degree of pain relief one may anticipate is uncertain.

Arachnoiditis, Epidural Scar Tissue, and Discitis

Scar tissue (arachnoiditis or epidural fibrosis) and discitis are nonmechanical causes of recurrent pain in the multiply operated back patient. Although the causes and specific locations of these lesions are different, they are discussed in the same section because none will respond to another surgical procedure.

Postoperative scar tissue formation can be divided into two main types based on anatomic location. Scar tissue that occurs beneath the dura is commonly referred to as *arachnoiditis.* Scar tissue can also form extradurally, either directly on the cauda equina or around the nerve root.

Arachnoiditis is strictly defined as an inflammation of the pia-arachnoid membrane surrounding the spinal cord or cauda equina. The condition may be present in varying degrees of severity, from mild thickening of the membranes to solid adhesions. The scarring may be severe enough to obliterate the subarachnoid space and block the flow of contrast agents.

The cause of this condition has been attributed to many factors; lumbar spine surgery and previous injections of contrast material seem to be the most frequent precipitating factors. Oil-base dye, formerly used in myelography, is highly associated with the occurrence of arachnoiditis. Postoperative infection may also play a role in the pathogenesis. The exact mechanism by which arachnoiditis develops from these events is not clear.

There is no uniform clinical presentation for arachnoiditis. The history often reveals more than one previous operation and a pain-free interval of between 1 and 6 mo. Often these patients will complain of back and leg pain. Physical examination is not conclusive; alterations in neurologic status may be on the basis of a previous operation. As mentioned earlier, myelography, CT, and MRI can be helpful in confirming the diagnosis.

At present no effective treatment is available for arachnoiditis. Surgical intervention has not proven effective in eliminating the scar tissue or significantly reducing the pain. Along with much needed encouragement, various nonoperative measures can be used. Epidural steroids, transcutaneous nerve stimulation, spinal cord stimulation, operant conditioning, bracing, and patient education have all been tried. None of these will lead to a cure, but when used judiciously they will provide symptomatic relief for varying periods. Patients should be detoxified from all narcotics, placed on amitriptyline (Elavil), and encouraged to do as much physical activity as possible. Treating these patients is a real challenge, and the physician must be willing to devote time and patience to achieve optimal results.

Formation of scar tissue outside the dura on the cauda equina or directly on nerve roots is a relatively common occurrence. This epidural scar tissue can act as a constrictive mass about the neural elements and may cause postoperative pain. However, although most patients have some epidural scar tissue, only an unpredictable few become symptomatic.

Patients with epidural scarring may present with symptoms at any time, from several months to a year after surgery. The onset is gradual, and they generally complain of back pain, leg pain, or both. Commonly, no neurologic findings are present but a positive tension sign may occur, purely on the basis of scar formation around a nerve root. The diagnosis is best differentiated from a recurrent herniated disc using gadolinium-enhanced MRI.

As with arachnoiditis, there is no definitive treatment for epidural scar tis-
sue. Prevention may be the best answer, and a free-fat graft or a piece of gel foam is often used as an interposition membrane to minimize scar tissue after laminectomy. Once scar tissue has formed, surgery is not successful because scarring will reform in even greater quantities. One doctor's scar is no better than another. The treatment program should be similar to that already described for arachnoiditis.

Discitis is an uncommon but debilitating complication of lumbar disc surgery. Its pathogenesis is postulated to be direct inoculation of the avascular disc space, but it is not completely understood. The onset of symptoms is usually 1 mo after surgery, and most patients will complain of severe back pain. Physical examination will sometimes reveal fever, a positive tension sign, and occasionally a superficial abscess.

If discitis is suspected from the history and physical examination, an erythrocyte sedimentation rate (ESR), blood cultures, and a plain radiograph should be obtained. Plain radiographs may not demonstrate the changes of disc space narrowing and endplate erosion in early stages. Contrast MRI may confirm the diagnosis.

Effective treatment has been controversial. It is recommended that the patient be placed at bed rest acutely with immobilization of the lumbar spine, with or without a brace or corset. If the patient experiences progressive pain after adequate immobilization or has constitutional symptoms, a needle aspiration should be performed. If a bacterial organism is identified, administration of 6 wk of intravenous antibiotics in indicated. There is no need for open disc space biopsy if the patient responds to conservative therapy. With improvement of symptoms (e.g., pain, ESR), the patient may ambulate as tolerated.

CONCLUSION

In conclusion, it should be stressed that the physician must take an organized approach to the evaluation of the multiply operated back patient. The origin of the problem in many cases is a faulty decision to perform the original surgical procedure. Further exploratory surgery is not warranted and will lead only to further disability. Another operative procedure is indicated only when objective findings for a specific diagnosis are present.

The cause of each patient's complaint must be accurately localized and identified. In addition to the spine specialist's evaluation, the patient's psychosocial and general medical status needs thorough investigation. Once the spine is identified as the source of the patient's symptoms, specific features should be sought in the patient's clinical history, physical examination, and radiographic studies. The number of previous operations, characteristics of the pain-free interval, and predominance of leg pain or back pain are the major historical points. The most important aspects of the physical examination are the neurologic findings and the presence of a tension sign. Plain radiographs, motion films, CT, and MRI all have specific roles in the work-up. When all the information is integrated, the physician usually can separate the patients with arachnoiditis, epidural scar tissue, and discitis from those with mechanical problems of the spine.

SUGGESTED READING

1. Borenstein DG, Wiesel SW. *Low back pain: medical diagnosis and comprehensive management.* Philadelphia: WB Saunders; 1989.
2. Frymoyer JW, ed. *The adult spine: principles and practice.* New York: Raven Press; 1992.
3. Rothman RH, Simeone FA, eds. *The spine.* 3rd ed. Philadelphia: WB Saunders; 1992.
4. Weinstein JN, Wiesel SW, eds. *The lumbar spine from the International Society for the Study of the Lumbar Spine.* Philadelphia: WB Saunders; 1992.

9

Management of Syndromes Related to Herniated Discs

Edward N. Hanley, Jr.

*Department of Orthopaedic Surgery, Carolinas Medical Center,
Charlotte, North Carolina 28203, USA*

Key Points

- Neck pain is common; conservative treatment is usually successful.

- Cervical radiculopathy is usually caused by a disc herniation. Conservative treatment is generally successful; however, surgery is indicated if radicular pain is severe and persistent for more than 6 to 12 wk.

- Spinal cord compression and long-tract symptoms may be caused by a central cervical disc herniation; treatment is by anterior disc excision, bone grafting, and fusion.

- Lumbar disc herniation and sciatica are fairly common but are far less frequent than is idiopathic low back pain.

- Sciatica is usually due to lumbar disc herniation; the outcome is usually favorable.

- Surgery for lumbar disc herniation and sciatica is indicated if acute bladder and bowel impairment is present (cauda equina syndrome) or if sciatic pain is incapacitating and persistent for more than 6 to 12 wk.

- Confirmation of the clinical level of disc herniation must be made by imaging (CT and/or MRI).

- With proper patient selection, surgery for lumbar disc herniation and sciatica can be expected to lead to excellent results in the majority of patients.

Understanding of the etiology, appropriate historical data gathering, and expertise in the physical examination lead to a more accurate classification of patients and an objective determination of when and how to apply the various treatment modalities, including surgery. Such a careful evaluation can be expected to facilitate the chances of symptom improvement and functional recovery.

The most important aspect of surgical decision making is in the history. Impatient or inappropriate questioning often leads to improper patient symptom classification, which in turn may result in disappointing outcomes for both the patient and the surgeon. With proper organizational concepts, one should be able to achieve over 85% satisfactory results for patients in either the nonoperative or the operative group. The successful outcome of patients treated nonoperatively is primarily the result of the benign natural history of neck and low back–related disorders, whereas the satisfactory outcomes of surgery relate mostly to appropriate patient selection and meticulous surgical technique.

Unfortunately, we are intrinsically biased or "trained" to attempt to place patients into treatment categories for which we have something to do. For surgeons this is usually a surgical "solution." Surgeons must resist this temptation or otherwise be willing to find themselves labeled as "good intention" doctors with less than optimal surgical results. As emphasized previously, neck pain has little if anything to do with radicular arm/forearm pain and low back pain does not necessarily relate to radicular pain below the knee.

Successful surgical results most often relate to the response to one simple question: "What hurts more, your neck or your arm?" or "What hurts more, your back or your leg?" If the answer is neck or back pain, then almost always the patient and you are best served by nonoperative treatment. Despite anecdotal or limited literature to the contrary, successful results of surgical treatment for "idiopathic," undiagnosed, or "discogenic" neck or back pain is in the range of 30% to 50%, compared with 80% to 95% for neurocompressive lesions.

Other factors that may influence outcome include the age of the patient, compensation issues, smoking habit, psychosocial characteristics, and bone quality (osteoporosis).

NECK PAIN

Neck pain is a common complaint. Its onset is frequently preceded by a traumatic or perceived injury. It is believed to be caused by either muscular problems or changes within or around the intervertebral disc. Physical examination is generally unremarkable, with findings restricted to local tenderness and diminished range of motion. Although referred pain may be present, the neurologic examination is usually normal. Radiographic examination may reveal no abnormalities or may show the disc space narrowing and osteophyte formation typically found in most adults. Nonoperative measures are generally appropriate. These include short-term rest, immobilization with a collar, heat or cold application, cervical traction, and nonsteroidal anti-inflammatory agents.

Manipulative therapy and trigger point or facet injections are rarely indicated. Diagnostic imaging (CT, MRI, myelography) is not indicated in such conditions as little is added to the therapeutic decision-making process and "abnormal findings" can potentially lead to inappropriate therapeutic decision making (see Chapter 6). Surgical treatment for this condition is controversial, as is diagnostic discography. Although anterior disc excision and fusion has been advocated by some for treatment of this condition, surgical results are most often less than satisfactory and must be compared to the natural history of this process.

Cervical Disc Herniation

The pathogenesis of degeneration of a cervical intervertebral disc is no different from that associated with the lumbar spine. It is epitomized by dehydration, fibrosis, and ultimately mechanical incompetence of the disc. It is progressive with age, and by middle life most individuals will show radiographic evidence of cervical spondylosis.

Symptomatic patients may present with neck pain, referred axial/shoulder pain, radiculopathy, or, on occasion, myelopathy as a result of the above-described process. Some may be genetically predisposed, and other problems may be related to mechanical or biochemical aberrations superimposed on the "normal" aging process. As in the lumbar spine, psychosocial, lifestyle, or work-related issues may exacerbate symptoms or cloud the picture.

Other disease states or conditions may mimic cervical disc disease and lead to confusion in the diagnosis. These include tumorous conditions (cervical intraspinal and extraspinal, brain, and shoulder girdle lesions); entrapment syndromes of the upper extremity (thoracic outlet and peripheral nerve syndromes); afflictions of the shoulder (rotator cuff tendinitis, bursitis, impingement syndromes); or even angina. These conditions must be considered in the differential diagnosis of neck or neck/upper extremity symptoms, particularly in older patients.

Cervical Radiculopathy

Cervical disc herniation occurs relatively frequently and can cause radicular symptoms and/or spinal cord compression if there is impingement of a cervical nerve root as it exits off the spinal cord through the cervical foramen or the spinal cord itself. Symptoms are usually limited to one dermatome or sclerotome but, due to vagaries of rootlet exit, overlap may occur. Disc herniations occur most commonly at the most mobile segments of the neck: C5-6, followed by C6-7 and C4-5. These intervertebral levels are also the most commonly noted to exhibit degenerative changes by radiographs and imaging studies. Disc herniations or foraminal encroachment by osteophytes typically involve the nerve root exiting at the level of the herniation as opposed to in the lumbar spine, where the nerve root crossing the narrowed area exits one level below (e.g., C6 root for C5-6 herniation and L5 root for L4-5 herniation). Extrusion and migration of a disc are less common than in the lumbar spine, but symptomatic central protrusions seem to be more common and are likely to cause more global symptoms. These occurrences are probably related to the anatomy of the region (smaller canal, presence of spinal cord). Cervical spinal cord compression due to central disc protrusion may cause muscle weakness, paresthesia, and pain, both in the legs and in the arms, depending on the exact location of the protrusion.

The symptoms and findings related to nerve root dysfunction from a herniated cervical disc have been well delineated. Pain and a sensation of numbness are the most common symptoms; motor weakness of a mild degree is often present, and reflex changes are a less reliable sign. Muscle atrophy is rare. Headaches, facial pain, and chest and shoulder girdle pain may confuse the issue.

Conservative Measures

Initial treatment is similar to that for patients with spondylotic or idiopathic neck pain and includes rest, the application of a soft collar, and medication with nonsteroidal anti-inflammatory drugs (NSAIDs) or analgesics and, on occasion, muscle relaxants. Recently, epidural steroid injection in the cervical region has been shown to be of some benefit in certain instances. However, complications from this technique can occur and caution should be exercised. In the case of acute disc herniation in the cervical spine with nerve root and/or spinal cord involvement, manipulation should be avoided.

The Selection of Patients for Cervical Disc Surgery

The majority of patients respond to nonoperative measures, and symptoms and neurologic deficits will improve over a period of several weeks. If major neurologic deficit exists, as in the case of spinal cord compression, or if radicular symptoms exist and are incapacitating over a period of 6 to 12 wk, further diagnostic evaluation and surgical consideration may be appropriate. Myelography/CT or MRI evaluation each has its advocates. It is essential, however, that the findings of these studies correlate precisely with the patient's symptoms and clinical findings before a surgical procedure is undertaken.

Operative intervention consists of anterior disc excision, anterior disc excision and interbody fusion, or posterior foraminotomy with or without disc excision. Orthopaedic surgeons have generally favored anterior disc excision and fusion. This may be combined with disc fragment excision and osteophyte removal or alternatively disc excision alone and interbody fusion. It is believed that with fusion, which provides maintenance of disc space height and stability, the spondylotic osteophytes will resorb over time, thus facilitating nerve root decompression. Recently, operative decompression of the nerve root has become more common. Although disc excision without fusion has been advocated by some, this is generally not favored. Posterior laminotomy/foraminotomy is generally reserved for patients with foraminal discs or primary osteophytic disease. Anterior disc excision and fusion is the most appropriate procedure for most patients with central disc herniation associated with spinal cord and nerve root compression.

Surgery for Cervical Disc Herniation

The approach is anterior (i.e., with the patient in the supine position). The anterior part of the cervical spine is surgically exposed, usually on the left side of the trachea (Figs. 1 and 2). The intervertebral disc in question is excised in toto, and disc fragments that may be present in the spinal canal or intervertebral foramen are removed. The procedure is usually performed with magnification loupes with a headlight or with an operative microscope. A bone graft is obtained from the iliac crest and placed within the evac-

uated intervertebral space (Fig. 3). In selected cases, the use of internal fixation has been advocated by some authors. This consists of a plate that is fixed by screws to the anterior side of the vertebrae above and below the bone graft. Postoperatively a cervical collar is usually worn for about 6 wk. Anterior cervical disc excision is generally a safe procedure with very few neurologic complications and with a high probability of relief of symptoms.

LUMBAR DISC HERNIATION

The symptoms of sciatica due to nerve root compression most often relate to aberrations of the lumbar intervertebral disc. This has led to widespread surgical treatment of this condition and a gradual

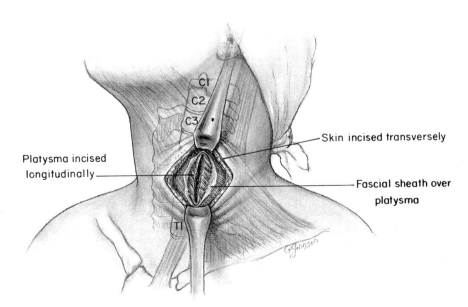

FIG. 1. Anterior approach to the cervical spine. (From Wood and Hanley (1992), with permission.)

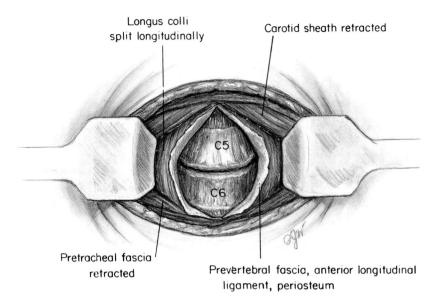

FIG. 2. Exposure and delineation of the anterior cervical spine. (From Wood and Hanley (1992), with permission.)

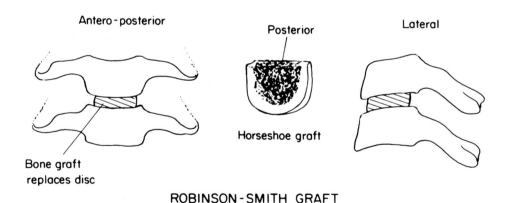

ROBINSON - SMITH GRAFT

FIG. 3. Bone graft placement after cervical disc excision. Some prefer to place the cortical portion of the graft posterior to minimize graft collapse. (From Wood and Hanley (1992), with permission.)

expansion of surgical indications for it and related conditions. In recent years we have attempted to look objectively at the outcome of such intervention and to determine which factors influence success or failure. Along with this we are beginning to accrue information on our ability accurately to diagnose other conditions affecting the lumbar spine and to gain insight into their natural history.

Although frequently lumped together in discussions and analyses, there are vast differences between the problems of low back pain and those of sciatica. The magnitude of low back pain in terms of incidence and prevalence, diagnosis and treatment perplexity, impairment, disability, and cost to society towers over the reasonably well-defined entity of sciatica due to a herniated intervertebral disc.

From available information it seems that the lifetime prevalence of low back pain approximates 60% to 80%, with longstanding low back pain problems in roughly 10% to 20% of the population. Each year 2% to 5% of adults will visit a physician for time lost from work due to low back pain. The societal costs for low back pain related to medical care and disability are enormous, estimated to exceed $50 billion annually.

The lifetime prevalence of a herniated disc seems to be in the vicinity of 2%, a small fraction of that of low back pain. Determination of the cost related to herniated discs is difficult, but it is reasonable to assume that at least some of it is included in that attributed to low back pain conditions, particularly for individuals for whom interventional therapy has failed.

The natural history of sciatica is predominantly that of spontaneous improvement. If we look at the lifetime prevalence of the disease in those patients with sciatica or those who have persistent radiculopathy (10% to 25%), less than 0.5% of the population should come to consideration of surgical treatment for such a condition. This, however, is not the case. In the United States the lifetime prevalence for spine surgery seems to be 3% to 4%, compared to only 1% in Scandinavia. There are numerous regional variations in rates of disc surgery in the United States. The absolute reasons for this are unclear, but it seems that the number of surgeons trained to perform such procedures and philosophical variations may influence how often such operations are performed. Although the indications for surgery seem to be quite clear-cut, they are not as standardized or agreed upon as one would like.

Conservative Measures

Scientific analysis has revealed that only brief periods of bed rest and specific back school programs are efficacious in the nonoperative treatment of the herniated disc. Nonsteroidal anti-inflammatory medications have been implicated as effective by some nonrandomized trials. Epidural steroids may on occasion be beneficial. Most patients with disc herniation and radiculopathy will have a successful outcome when treated nonoperatively, and this may or may not correlate with disc fragment resorption.

Although a vast array of nonsurgical treatment modalities exist (braces, heat, ice, biofeedback, traction, manipulation, massage, oral steroids, acupuncture, psychologic support, etc.), there remains no true scientifically valid evidence that such methods improve the natural history of the problem. However, just because such treatment methods have not been validated as improving on the natural history of the problem, one cannot assume that they are not helpful or that they are harmful.

The Selection of Patients for Lumbar Disc Surgery

Long-term studies (4 to 10 yr) comparing operative and nonoperative treatment for patients with mild radiculopathy show no statistically significant difference in outcome. Thus, in cases of mild radiculopathy, the only real benefit from surgery for most patients is quicker relief from their sciatic pain. The treating physician should inform patients about these facts. One should select for surgery those patients for whom nonop-

erative measures have failed or will probably fail and who can be reasonably expected to have symptomatic relief and to experience a return to relatively normal function after such a procedure. In the past, five clinical criteria had been used to select surgical candidates: (a) impairment of bladder or bowel function, (b) gross motor weakness, (c) evidence of increasing impairment of neural function, (d) severe persistent sciatic pain, and (e) recurrent episodes of sciatica. At present these indications, other than the impairment of bladder or bowel function and major motor deficit, would be considered relative. Thus, the usual indication for surgery is pain, and clearly the decision to undertake surgery is influenced by the patient's desires and needs and by the opinion of the evaluating surgeon. Thus, it is essential to have an accurate clinical diagnosis of the cause of sci-

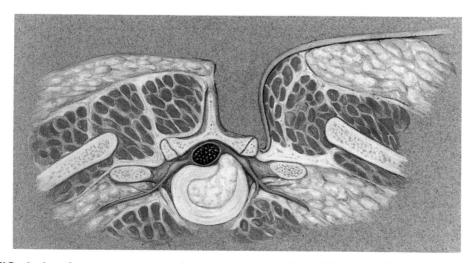

FIG. 4. Laminotomy exposure for disc excision. (From Wood and Hanley (1991), with permission.)

atica, an anatomic level of the lesion, and support for both by appropriate imaging investigations (CT/MRI).

Prolonged symptoms (>3 to 6 mo), abnormal illness (pain) behavior, a compensation work situation, cigarette smoking, and an age over 40 may contribute to a negative surgical outcome and should also be taken into consideration, particularly if more than one of these factors is present. By far the most common cause of treatment failure is poor patient selection.

Surgery for Lumbar Disc Herniation

The surgery can be performed under spinal anesthesia, but usually general anesthesia is recommended. The patient is positioned on the operating table on a special positioning frame that allows the abdomen to hang free without compression of the vena cava, thus minimizing epidural venous stasis. Such positioning has been shown to reduce intraoperative bleeding markedly during spinal surgery. Blood loss per se may not be a problem in lumbar disc surgery, but minimizing bleeding makes the surgical dissection more exact. The relevant part of the lumbar spine is exposed through a midline incision, and the involved motion segment is verified by an intraoperative x-ray film. Paraspinal muscles on the symptomatic side are dissected free and retracted (Fig. 4). A small laminotomy is then performed, and the ligamentum flavum is sharply excised or reflected. As in cervical spinal surgery, the procedure is usually performed under magnification with loupes and headlight or with an operating microscope. The nerve root is visualized and, if necessary, carefully retracted medially to allow exposure and removal of the disc herniation and of associated free fragments that may be present in the epidural space (Fig. 5). Postoperatively the patient is encouraged to be out of bed and to ambulate as soon as possible after recovery from anesthesia. The hospital stay is usually short (1 to 4 days). Sitting on low chairs, car driving, excessive lifting, and forward bending are usually restricted for 3 to 6 wk. Return to work generally takes place during the same postoperative time frame. In properly selected patients, excision of a herniated disc for relief of sciatica should provide rapid relief of symptoms in over 90% of patients. Relief of back pain is far less predictable. Recurrent disc herniation may occur in 5% to 10%. The results of reoperation for such a recurrence at the same level and site are in general less successful. Complications in terms of discitis, dural tears, nerve root injuries, and iliac vessel penetration (due to anterior disc space penetration) are rare.

Alternative Treatment Techniques

Percutaneous procedures have in the last decade been proposed as a relatively noninvasive method of treating lumbar disc problems. These include mechanical suction discectomy, laser ablative discectomy, and arthroscopic techniques. Unfortunately, recent clinical experience indicates that the rates of a successful result are not as high as those reported for open discectomy, with success rates ranging from 50% to 80%. These results are similar to those reported for chymopapain in the 1970s and 1980s. Crit-

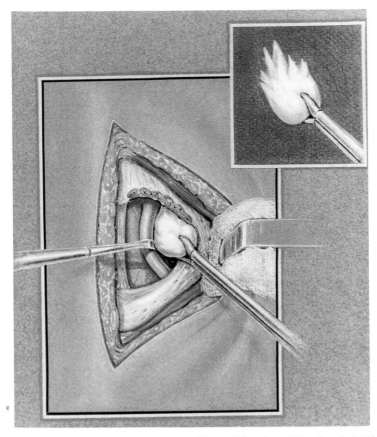

FIG. 5. Method of disc fragment excision. (From Wood and Hanley (1991), with permission.)

ics of these techniques suggest that poor results are primarily related to inappropriate expansion of surgical indications.

SUGGESTED READING

Cervical Disc Herniation

1. Boden SD, McCowin PR, Davis DO. Abnormal magnetic-resonance imaging scans of the lumbar spine in asymptomatic subjects: a prospective investigation. *J Bone Joint Surg [Am]* 1990;72A:1178–1184.

2. Clements DH, O'Leary PF. Anterior cervical discectomy and fusion. *Spine* 1990;15:1023–1025.

3. Gore DR, Sepic SB, Gardner GM. Neck pain: a long term follow up of 205 patients. *Spine* 1987;12:1–5.

4. Herkowitz HN. A comparison of anterior cervical fusion, cervical laminectomy, and cervical laminoplasty for the surgical management of multiple level spondylotic radiculopathy. *Spine* 1988;13:774–780.

5. Herkowitz HN, Kurz LT, Overhotz DP. Surgical management of cervical soft disc herniation: a comparison between anterior and posterior approach. *Spine* 1990;15:1026–1030.

6. Lunsford L, Bissonette D, Janetta P. Anterior surgery for cervical disc disease: Part I. *J Neurosurg* 1980;53:1–11.
7. Whitecloud TS, Seago RA. Cervical discogenic syndrome: results of operative intervention in patients with positive discography. *Spine* 1987;12:313–316.
8. Wiesel SW, Herkowitz HN, eds. Cervical disc disease. *Semin Spine Surg* 1989;1(4).
9. Wood EG, Hanley EN Jr. Types of anterior cervical grafts. *Orthop Clin North Am* 1992; 23:475–486.

Lumbar Disc Herniation

10. Boden SD, Davis DO, Dina TS, Patronas JJ, Wiesel SW. Abnormal magnetic-resonance imaging scans of the lumbar spine in asymptomatic subjects: a prospective investigation. *J Bone Joint Surg [Am]* 1990;72A:403–408.
11. Hanley EN Jr. The cost of surgical intervention for lumbar disc herniation. In: Weinstein JN, ed. *Clinical efficacy and outcome in the diagnosis and treatment of low back pain.* New York: Raven Press; 1992:125–133.
12. Hanley EN Jr, Shapiro DE. The development of low back pain after excision of a lumbar disc. *J Bone Joint Surg [Am]* 1989;71A: 719–721.
13. Saal JA, Saal JS, Herlog RJ. The natural history of lumbar disc extrusions treated nonoperatively. *Spine* 1990;15:683–686.
14. Spengler DM, Freeman CW. Patient selection for lumbar discectomy: an objective approach. *Spine* 1979;4:129–134.
15. Weber H. Lumbar disc herniation: a controlled prospective study with ten years of observation. *Spine* 1983;8:131–140.
16. Wiesel SW, Bell GR, eds. Lumbar disc disease. *Semin Spine Surg* 1989;1(1).
17. Wood EG, Hanley EN Jr. Lumbar disc herniation and open limited discectomy: indications, techniques, and results. *Operative Techniques Orthopaedics* 1991;1(1):23–28.

10

Management of Syndromes Related to Spinal Stenosis

Harry N. Herkowitz

Department of Orthopaedic Surgery, William Beaumont Hospital, Royal Oak, Michigan 48073, USA

Key Points ━━━━━━━━━━━━━━━━━━━━━━━━━━━

- Spinal stenosis is most common in elderly patients and is defined as narrowing of the spinal canal and/or lateral nerve root canals.

- The underlying processes leading to spinal stenosis are degenerative changes in facet joints and intervertebral discs and buckling of the ligamentum flavum.

- Spinal stenosis can occur in both the cervical and the lumbar spine.

- Surgical treatment includes decompressive laminectomy and sometimes fusion.

Spinal stenosis in the cervical or lumbar region may result in mechanical compression of the spinal cord and/or nerve roots. The development of symptoms is usually more gradual and slow than in the case of disc herniation. The patients with stenosis-related syndromes are also generally older than the patients with disc herniation. This means that there are often other medical conditions involved which may influence the management of these older patients.

The underlying pathologic reactions of the spine that may lead to stenosis are degenerative changes in the intervertebral discs and the facet joints, including buckling of the ligamentum flavum. An understanding of these changes is essential for correct diagnosis and treatment of spinal stenosis-related syndromes.

CERVICAL SPINAL STENOSIS

Neck pain associated with cervical spinal stenosis usually mimics the underlying degenerative changes that are often present in this patient population. These symptoms include paraspinal discomfort, occipital radiation, scapular radiation, and referred pain to the deltoid region. These symptoms wax and wane and are usually more severe during the daytime hours when the patient is active.

Arm pain in a dermatomal distribution occurs with nerve root entrapment, usually secondary to the degenerative changes that are present in association with the narrow spinal canal. As in cervical disc herniation, the most common level of involvement is C5-6, followed by C6-7. The radicular pattern may be unilateral or bilateral and may be accompanied by weakness in that specific dermatomal distribution, in addition to the arm pain (Table 1).

Symptoms and signs of true spinal cord compression occur when the degenerative osteophytes impinge on the spinal cord in association with the already narrow spinal canal. These changes will occur usually when the spinal canal is narrowed less than 12 mm since the normal spinal canal measures anywhere from 12 to 22 mm in diameter. In addition, the C5-6 level has the widest spinal cord diameter with the narrowest spinal canal space and therefore is the segment most predisposed to developing myelopathic changes.

TABLE 1. *Cervical radiculopathy symptoms and findings*

Disk level	Nerve root	Symptoms and findings
C2-3	C3	*Pain:* Back of neck, mastoid process, pinna of ear *Sensory change:* Back of neck, mastoid process, pinna of ear *Motor deficit:* None readily detectable except by EMG *Reflex change:* None
C3-4	C4	*Pain:* Back of neck, levator scapulae, anterior chest *Sensory change:* Back of neck, levator scapulae, anterior chest *Motor deficit:* None readily detectable except by EMG *Reflex change:* None
C4-5	C5	*Pain:* Neck, tip of shoulder, anterior arm *Sensory change:* Deltoid area *Motor deficit:* Deltoid, biceps *Reflex change:* Biceps
C5-6	C6	*Pain:* Neck, shoulder, medial border of scapula, lateral arm, dorsal forearm *Sensory change:* Thumb and index finger *Motor deficit:* Biceps *Reflex change:* Biceps
C6-7	C7	*Pain:* Neck, shoulder, medial border of scapula, lateral arm, dorsal forearm *Sensory change:* Index and middle fingers *Motor deficit:* Triceps *Reflex change:* Triceps
C7-T1	C8	*Pain:* Neck, medial border of scapula, medial aspect of arm and forearm *Sensory change:* Ring and little fingers *Motor deficit:* Intrinsic muscles of hand *Reflex change:* None

Several myelopathic syndromes may be produced, depending on which portion of the spinal cord is most affected. The transverse lesion syndrome is due to involvement of the posterior columns and the spinal thalamic and corticospinal tracts. These patients present with diffuse weakness below the level of the cord compression. The motor syndrome is due to cortical spinal tract involvement and produces upper and lower extremity weakness with predominant arm involvement. A Brown-Séquard syndrome is associated with ipsilateral paralysis and contralateral loss of pain and temperature sensation due to the compression of the lateral cortical spinal tract. It has the best prognosis of the spinal cord syndromes.

These cord syndromes may develop along three different tracks. They may be sudden in onset with progressive deterioration, which is extremely uncommon. They may develop insidiously with a gradual deterioration of symptoms and function, which is the second most common form of presentation. The most common concept is an insidious cyclical pattern of active symptoms followed by quiescent periods of no progression.

The physical examination of the patient with radiculopathy should include motion evaluation of the cervical spine and maneuvers to reproduce arm pain such as the Sperling maneuver, which is extension, lateral flexion to the side of the complaint, and axial loading on the head, which should reproduce the radicular pain. In addition, weakness in the specific nerve root distribution affected may be present. It is important to rule out intrinsic shoulder abnormality and peripheral nerve root entrapment syndromes, such as carpal tunnel, anterior interosseous nerve compression, or ulnar nerve entrapment at the elbow as a cause of the patient's arm complaints.

The most common presenting complaint of patients with myelopathy is a change in their walking pattern. These patients often complain of a feeling of imbalance or a lack of coordination when they attempt to ambulate. Complaints of bowel and bladder dysfunction are usually late in onset, as are posterior column findings. The physical examination will usually reveal a combination of weakness, hyperreflexia, and spasticity depending on which cord syndrome is present. Specific reflex testing including Hoffman's reflex, the inverted radial reflex, and Babinski's sign should be checked. It is important to rule out intrinsic spinal cord pathologic conditions such as tumors, demyelinating diseases, or syringomyelia as the cause of the patient's complaints. In addition, it is important to rule out lesions above the foramen magnum, which can be done with a careful facial examination and the jaw jerk.

Conservative Treatment

Neck Pain

Nonoperative treatment of neck pain consists of limited immobilization using a soft collar, aspirin or nonsteroidal anti-inflammatory drugs, and a limited use of moist heat to the affected areas. In most cases, symptoms will subside within 10 days to 3 wk.

Radiculopathy

Most patients with radiculopathy will respond to simple measures of neck

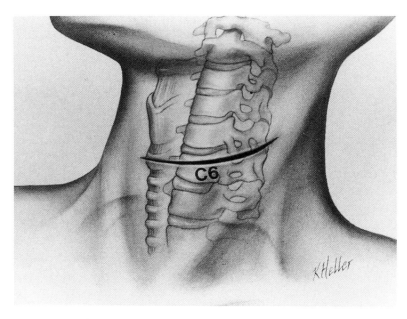

FIG. 1. Schematic of cervical spine demonstrating the incision used for anterior fusion.

immobilization with a soft collar, aspirin, or nonsteroidal anti-inflammatory drugs. If symptoms do not abate, consideration may be given to a limited course of outpatient physical therapy consisting of intermittent cervical traction, ultrasound, and heat along with soft tissue massage in conjunction with isometric neck strengthening exercise. From 85% to 90% of patients will respond to this regime.

Myelopathy

Patients with myelopathy may be followed nonoperatively as long as progression of their disease does not interfere with their lifestyle. In other words, patients with mild symptoms and signs who are functioning reasonably well may be observed before recommending sur-

gical intervention. For patients with progressive deterioration of neurologic function and progressive limitations of ability to ambulate, nonoperative treatment is not recommended.

Surgery

Most patients with these syndromes respond to nonoperative management. There is, however, a small percentage of patients for whom surgery is indicated (10% to 20%). The indications for surgery in patients with radiculopathy are (a) persistent or recurring arm pain despite an adequate trial of nonoperative treatment (6 wk to 3 mo), (b) progressive neurologic deficit, and (c) significant alteration of quality of life. The indications for surgery in patients with myelopathy are

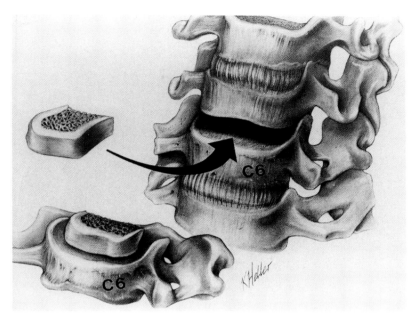

FIG. 2. Schematic of anterior cervical spine showing insertion of horseshoe-shaped bone graft after discectomy.

progressive neurologic deficit or the inability to care for themselves adequately.

Radiculopathy

Anterior discectomy with fusion is the gold standard operative treatment for cervical stenosis causing radiculopathy at one to two interspaces. The affected interspace is entered from a left-sided anterior approach centered over a transverse incision at the midpoint of the sternocleidomastoid muscle (Fig. 1). The anterovertebral disc is completely excised, after which a horseshoe-shaped wedge of bone taken from the patient's iliac crest is inserted into the disc space (Fig. 2). No attempt is made to excise any posterior osteophytes when radiculopathy only is present.

Anterior discectomy without bony fusion has not been shown to be effective and is not recommended. When diffuse stenosis is present with compression behind the vertebral body, a corpectomy is necessary followed by a larger bone graft. *Corpectomy* refers to removing all or a portion of the vertebral body along with the disc. The bone grafting is either from iliac crest or the fibula (Fig. 3). This is most often indicated for patients with myelopathy.

For patients with radiculopathy the expected good outcome is 80% to 95%. In myelopathy, improvement rates are from 75% to 85% but are much less predictable than that of radiculopathy. Often one can expect only to deter further progression of the disease process. The most common complications of surgery are

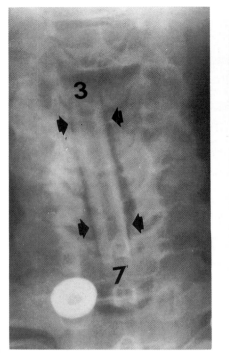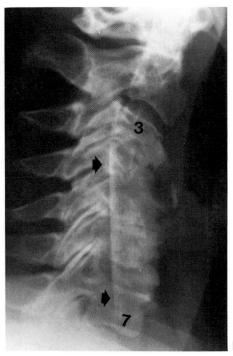

A   **B**

FIG. 3. AP **(A)** and lateral **(B)** radiographs showing fibular strut graft from C3-7 after multiple level corpectomies for cervical spinal stenosis.

pseudarthrosis (one-level fusion, 5% to 10%; two-level fusion, 10% to 20%; three-level fusion, 15% to 30%), dislodgement of the bone graft (1% to 2%), nerve injuries (1% to 2%), and graft site pain and/or numbness (10%).

Instrumentation

Anterior cervical plating has been advocated as an adjunct to anterior fusion (Fig. 4). To date, no study has substantiated and improved the fusion rate. Its present use in degenerative cervical stenosis has been confined to patients in whom a cervical corpectomy followed by a large bone graft has been performed. The anterior plate is added in lieu of placing a halo brace. Further studies are necessary before its use can be recommended generally.

Posterior Procedures

The posterior procedures include laminotomy, foraminotomy, laminectomy, and laminoplasty. *Laminotomy* refers to the removal of a small portion of the lamina and facet joint to decompress the cervical nerve root (Fig. 5). It is recommended for unilateral, single-level nerve compression. The long-term results are

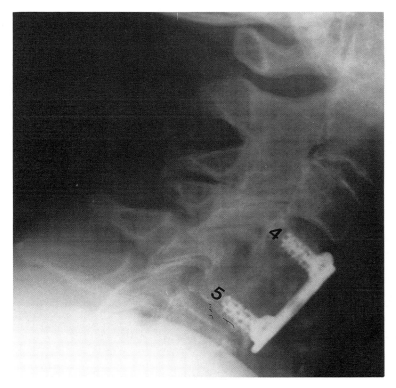

FIG. 4. Lateral cervical radiograph showing anterior cervical plate after C4-5 interbody fusion.

not as good as those of anterior discectomy and interbody fusion.

Laminectomy is a removal of the lamina(s) and usually a portion of the facet joint(s) (Fig. 6). It is most often used for multiple level radiculopathy or myelopathy. If too much of the facet joint is excised (greater than 25% bilaterally), this may lead to bony instability and persistent or recurrent pain and weakness (Fig. 7). The results of laminectomy are also inferior to those of anterior decompression and fusion.

Laminoplasty is a canal-expanding procedure that preserves the stability of

the cervical spine (Fig. 8). It is most often used for multilevel cervical stenosis with myelopathy and/or radiculopathy. It was first described by several authors in the early 1970s for patients with cervical myelopathy due to ossification of the posterior longitudinal ligament. The reported results are better than those of laminectomy for relief of symptoms and preservation of stability.

The complications of laminectomy include postlaminectomy kyphosis (i.e., the loss of the normal cervical lordosis leading to subluxation or kyphosis). This may lead to persistent or recurrent pain

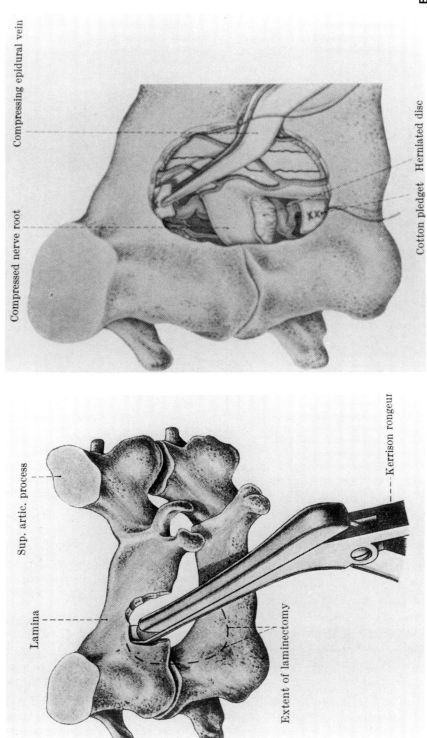

Sup. artic. process

Lamina

Extent of laminectomy

Kerrison rongeur

A

Compressing epidural vein

Compressed nerve root

Cotton pledget   Herniated disc

B

Fig. 5. A: Schematic of posterior cervical spine showing Kerrison rongeur developing the laminotomy–foraminotomy. **B:** Schematic showing completed foraminotomy with exposed nerve root and herniated disc beneath it.

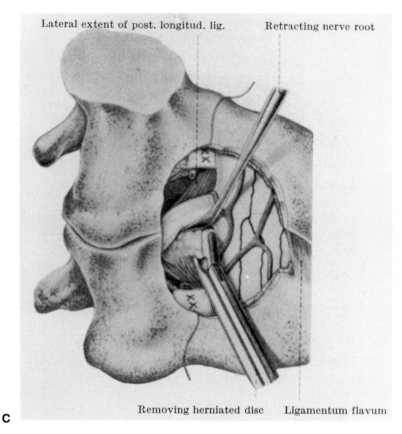

FIG. 5. *(Continued).* **C:** Schematic showing cervical nerve root being retracted and herniated disc being removed with pituitary rongeur.

and/or weakness requiring reconstructive surgery. The incidence of this complication in adults ranges from 5% to 40%. Laminoplasty, on the other hand, has been shown to be biomechanically superior to laminectomy and is the preferred posterior procedure for multiple level (three or more) disease. Kyphosis after laminoplasty is very rare.

In summary, cervical stenosis may lead to the development of radiculopathy and/or myelopathy. The majority of patients respond to nonoperative management. Surgical intervention has been shown to be safe and effective when nonoperative treatment fails.

LUMBAR SPINAL STENOSIS

Back pain associated with degenerated lumbar spinal stenosis is usually due to the degenerative arthritic changes that are present in this aged population. Due to its degenerative nature, back pain is usu-

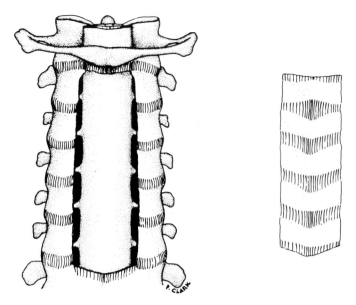

FIG. 6. Schematic of multiple level cervical laminectomy showing extent of decompression.

ally of a mechanical nature that is activity related. Severe rest pain or pain occurring at night should alert the physician to other causes, such as tumor or aneurysm.

Leg symptoms associated with spinal stenosis are of two varieties; they may be radicular, that is, following a specific dermatomal pattern similar to the symptoms of a herniated lumbar disc. Or they may be diffuse in origin, representing the condition of neurogenic claudication. Pains associated with neurogenic claudication are diffuse and nondermatomal, involve one or both lower extremities, and are activity related. They must be differentiated from vascular claudication since, in this elderly population, arterial insufficiency is common. The symptoms of neurogenic claudication are usually due to cauda equina compression from the thickened ligamentum flavum and hypertrophied

facet joints, whereas radicular pain associated with this condition is most often due to nerve entrapment in the lateral recess.

The compression of the cauda equina in spinal stenosis differs from the true cauda equina syndrome due to a central disc herniation. The symptoms of the true cauda equina syndrome are buttock hyperesthesia, progressive lower extremity weakness, and loss of bladder control. This syndrome is rare.

The symptoms associated with spinal stenosis usually run a course of intermittent episodes with periods of quiescence. Rarely do patients have progressive deterioration of function.

Conservative Treatment

Nonoperative treatment associated with spinal stenosis consists of restrict-

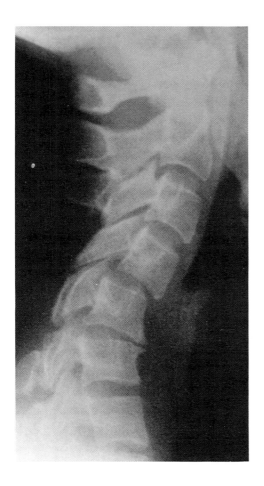

FIG. 7. Lateral cervical radiograph showing development of kyphosis after a C3-6 laminectomy.

ing activity and avoiding those maneuvers that reproduce pain. These are most commonly extension maneuvers or repetitive lifting and bending activity. In addition, for acute severe pain patients are placed at bed rest for 1 to 3 days. Longer periods may lead to atrophy and increased risk of deep vein thrombosis/pulmonary embolus. Aspirin remains the primary medication with nonsteroidal anti-inflammatory drugs as a backup. Muscle relaxants do not benefit patients with spinal stenosis.

Physical therapy in the form of massage, ultrasound, and moist heat may reduce the initial low back symptoms. Intermittent pelvic traction benefits some patients; however, no scientific evidence demonstrates a stenosis-reducing affect of traction. A lumbar corset provides abdominal support, restricts bending, and reminds the patient to be cautious. It is often helpful in the acute setting for 2 to 4 wk. Exercise should begin when pain abates. Isometric flexion exercises are beneficial. Extension exercises often

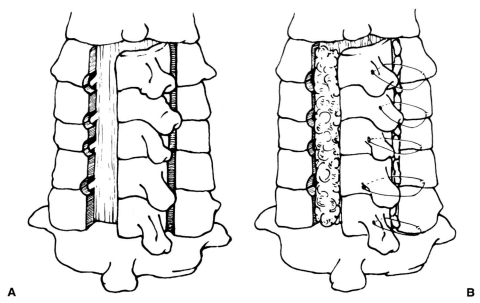

FIG. 8. A: Schematic demonstrating open door laminoplasty. **B:** Schematic demonstrating completed laminoplasty with lamina held open by multiple sutures and fat placed over exposed dura.

exacerbate stenotic symptoms. General aerobic conditioning is important and consists of walking, biking, or swimming exercise every other day for 20 to 30 min. This helps in overall conditioning and in weight reduction. Progressive resistance exercise is recommended but in older patients may not be realistic.

Surgery

If no response to nonoperative treatment occurs, surgical intervention is recommended in the following situations:

1. Failure to respond to nonoperative treatment (3-mo minimum)

2. Progressive neurologic deficit

3. Static neurologic deficit with persistent leg pain

4. Poor quality of life

Surgery is performed for leg pain, *not back pain alone.* Imaging studies are necessary to confirm stenosis and define significant levels of compression before proceeding with surgery. The standard operative procedure is decompressive lumbar laminectomy. It includes removal of the lamina and a portion of the facet joint(s) to decompress the dural sac and nerve roots (Fig. 9). The compression of the nerves is due to facet joint hypertrophy in combination with thickening of the ligamentum flavum, degeneration of the disc, and possibly subluxation of the vertebrae.

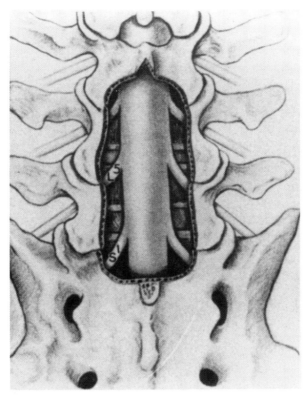

FIG. 9. Schematic demonstrating extent of decompressive laminectomy of L4-S1 with preservation of the facet joints.

The surgical success rate ranges from 60% to 70%. Approximately 10% to 20% of patients require further surgery due to stenosis at other lumbar levels, regrowth of the lamina, or the development of instability of the spine. The complications of surgery are those of any operative procedure in an older age group. The surgically specific complications are dural tear (5%), instability (5%), and nerve injury (1%).

There are several relative indications for a concomitant intertransverse process spinal fusion at the time of the decompressive laminectomy. These are based on preoperative and intraoperative structural alterations. The preoperative structural alterations are (a) degenerative spondylolisthesis with stenosis (Fig. 10), (b) scoliosis and/or kyphosis (Fig. 11), and (c) recurrent spinal stenosis at a previously decompressed level. The operative reasons necessitating fusion are (a) excessive removal of the facet joints (greater than 50% on each side) and (b) radical excision of the disc at the level of decompression.

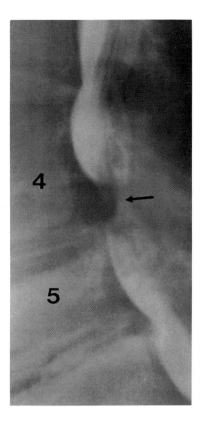

FIG. 10. Lateral lumbar myelogram of degenerative L4-5 spondylolisthesis (*arrow*) with spinal stenosis.

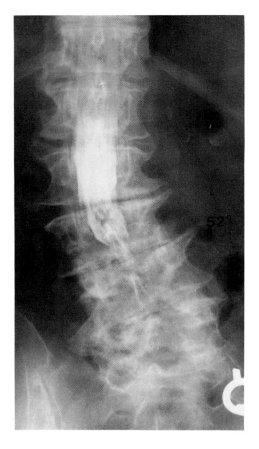

FIG. 11. AP radiograph showing scoliosis with spinal stenosis. The curvature was 50% correctable on side bending.

When is the addition of spinal instrumentation to the fusion necessary? The goals of internal fixation are (a) correction of deformity, (b) stabilization of the spine, (c) protection of the neural elements, (d) improvement of the fusion rate, (e) reduction of the number of segments requiring fusion, and (f) reduction of rehabilitation time. In view of these goals, the indications for instru-mentation after spinal stenosis decompression and arthrodesis are (a) correction of scoliosis and/or kyphosis, (b) arthrodesis of two or more motion segments, (c) recurrent spinal stenosis with iatrogenic spondylolisthesis, and (d) translational motion greater than 4 mm in flexion and extension (Fig. 12) and excessive angular motion (greater than 10° in flexion and extension).

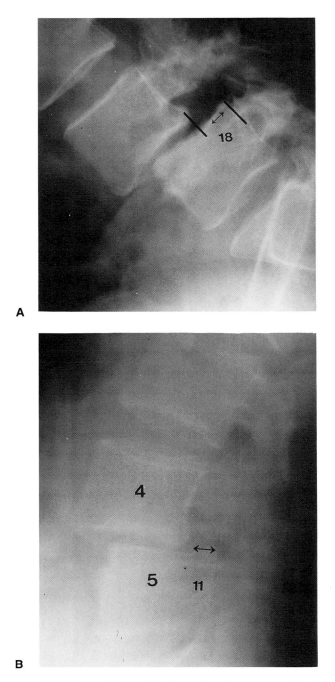

FIG. 12. A: Lateral flexion radiograph after prior decompressive laminectomy with 18 mm of forward motion at L4-5. **B:** Lateral extension radiograph showing reduction of the slippage to 11 mm.

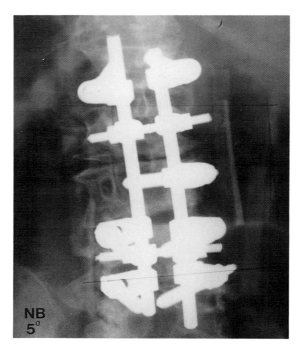

NB
5°

A

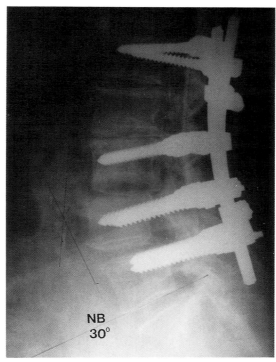

NB
30°

B

FIG. 13. A: AP radiograph demonstrating spinal instrumentation for 42° scoliosis corrected to 5° after three-level decompressive laminectomy. **B:** Lateral radiograph showing pedicle fixation of L1-2 with restoration of lumbar lordosis.

Instrumentation in older individuals presents unique considerations. The instrumentation system must address the lack of lamina, osteoporosis, and preservation of lumbar lordosis. At present, segmental pedicle fixation provides the optimal instrumentation system for degenerative lumbar disorder (Fig. 13). The role of pedicle fixation systems in the surgical treatment of lumbar spinal stenosis is an issue which needs further clinical research.

In summary, degenerative lumbar spinal stenosis presents with back and/or leg pains of varying severity and duration. Most patients lead a satisfactory lifestyle. For those patients who require surgery, the long-term results have been favorable and allow people to resume and maintain an active lifestyle.

SUGGESTED READING

Cervical Spine

1. Abitbol JJ, Garfin S. Surgical management of cervical disc disease: anterior cervical fusion. *Semin Spine Surg* 1989;1(4):233–238.
2. Bernhardt M, Hynes R, Blume H, White A. Cervical spondylotic myelopathy: current concepts review. *J Bone Joint Surg [Am]* 1993; 75A:119–129.
3. Boden S, McCowin P, Davis P, Dina T, Mark A, Wiesel S. Abnormal magnetic resonance scans of the cervical spine in asymptomatic subjects. *J Bone Joint Surg [Am]* 1990;72A: 1178–1184.
4. Bohlman H, Emery S, Goodfellow D, Jones P. Robinson anterior cervical discectomy and arthrodesis for cervical radiculopathy. *J Bone Joint Surg [Am]* 1993;75A:1298–1307.
5. Garfin SR, Herkowitz HN. The degenerative neck. *Orthop Clin North Am* 1992;23:3.
6. Herkowitz HN. The surgical management of cervical spondylotic radiculopathy and myelopathy. *Clin Orthop* 1989;239:94–108.
7. Nowinski G, Visarius H, Nolte L, Herkowitz H. A biomechanical comparison of cervical laminoplasty and cervical laminectomy with progressive facetectomy. *Spine* 1993;18: 1995–2004.
8. Robinson R, Walker A, Ferlic D. The results of anterior interbody fusion of the cervical spine. *J Bone Joint Surg [Am]* 1962;44A:1569–1587.

Lumbar Spine

9. Garfin S, Glover M, Booth R, et al. Laminectomy: a review of the Pennsylvania Hospital experience. *J Spin Dis* 1988;1:116–133.
10. Herkowitz HN, Kurz LT. Degenerative lumbar spondylolisthesis with spinal stenosis: a prospective study comparing decompression with decompression and intertransverse progressive arthrodesis. *J Bone Joint Surg [Am]* 1991;73A:802–808.
11. Herno A, Airaksinen O, Saari T. Long term results of surgical treatment of lumbar spinal stenosis. *Spine* 1993;18:1471–1474.
12. Herron L, Mangelsdorf C. Lumbar spinal stenosis: results of surgical treatment. *J Spin Dis* 1991;4:26–33.
13. Sanderson PL, Wood PL. Surgery for lumbar spinal stenosis in old people. *J Bone Joint Surg [Br]* 1993;75B:393–397.
14. Spengler D. Degenerative stenosis of the lumbar spine: current concepts review. *J Bone Joint Surg [Am]* 1987;69A:305–308.
15. Tile M, McNeil SR, Zarins RK, Pennal GF, Garside SH. Spinal stenosis: results of treatment. *Clin Orthop* 1976;115:104–108.

11

Deformities of the Spine

Stuart L. Weinstein

Department of Orthopaedic Surgery, University of Iowa Hospitals,
Iowa City, Iowa 52242, USA

Key Points

- The majority of patients with adolescent idiopathic scoliosis never require active treatment.

- Remaining growth potential and curve pattern and magnitude are the key prognostic factors in adolescent idiopathic scoliosis.

- In patients presenting for scoliosis with no known etiology, be very suspicious of rapid curve progression, early onset (younger than age 10), unusual curve patterns, or significant pain complaints. Further evaluation is mandatory.

- Back pain in children in contrast to adults is not common; it must be carefully evaluated.

- Congenital spine deformities cannot be treated by bracing.

- The normal thoracic kyphosis is between 20° and 45°.

- All radiographs to assess spondylolisthesis should be taken with the patient standing.

- Spondylolysis is an acquired condition.

- Less than 3% of all cases of herniated nucleus pulposus occur in children.

Spinal deformity generally occurs in either the coronal or sagittal plane or combinations thereof. Classification is based on the magnitude and the direction of the curvature, the location of its apex, and the cause. Spinal deformity may be associated with many conditions (Table 1).

GENERAL CONSIDERATIONS

The cause of the spinal deformity must be determined. Etiology determines natural history and, hence, dictates treatment. Etiology is determined by a history, physical exam, and appropriate imaging studies. Idiopathic scoliosis, the most common spinal deformity, is not a painful condition. Thus, any child who presents with scoliosis and pain must be examined for other spinal conditions that cause pain, such as Scheuermann kyphosis, tumors (spine and spinal cord), and spondylolisthesis and spondylolysis. Notation should be made as to how the deformity affects the patient and any physical limitations. Developmental milestones should be recorded. A careful family history must be obtained, seeking out any history of neurologic or congenital conditions that may be associated with the curvature.

Growth potential heavily influences treatment decisions; therefore, it must be

TABLE 1. *SRS (Scoliosis Research Society) classification of spine deformity*

SCOLIOSIS	Traumatic	Unilateral (unilateral
Idiopathic	Spinal muscular	unsegmented
Infantile (0–3 years)	atrophy	bar)
Resolving	Myelomeningocele	Bilateral (*bloc* verte-
Progressive	(paralytic)	brae)
Juvenile (4 years to	Dysautonomia (Riley-	Mixed
puberty onset)	Day)	Associated with neural
Adolescent (puberty	Other	tissue defect
onset to epiphyseal	Myopathic	Myelomeningocele
closure)	Arthrogryposis	Meningocele
Adult (epiphyses closed)	Muscular dystrophy	Spinal dysraphism
Neuromuscular	Duchenne (pseudo-	Diastematomyelia
Neuropathic	hypertrophic)	Other
Upper motor neuron	Limb-girdle	Neurofibromatosis
lesion	Facioscapulohumeral	Mesenchymal
Cerebral palsy	Congenital hypotonia	Marfan
Spinocerebellar	Myotonia dystrophics	Homocystinuria
degeneration	Other	Ehlers-Danlos
Friedreich	Congenital	Other
Charcot-Marie-Tooth	Failure of formation	Traumatic
Roussy-Lévy	Partial unilateral	Fracture or dislocation
Syringomyelia	(wedge vertebra)	(nonparalytic)
Spinal cord tumor	Complete unilateral	Postradiation
Spinal cord trauma	(hemivertebra)	Other
Other	Fully segmented	Soft tissue contractures
Lower motor neuron	Semisegmented	Postempyema
lesion	Nonsegmented	Burns
Poliomyelitis	Failure of segmentation	Other

carefully assessed. The development of secondary sex characteristics such as pubic hair, axillary hair, breast budding, and menarche should be noted. Details of any prior treatment should also be ascertained.

Each patient should have a complete physical and neurologic examination. Particular attention should be paid to the patient's body habitus and any evidence of congenital abnormalities. The skin should be inspected for nodules called *neurofibromas* or brownish patches called *café-au-lait spots* indicative of neurofibromatosis. The skin over the sacrum should be examined for evidence of hairy patches, dimpling, pigmentation changes, nevi, and lipomas, which may be associated with spinal dysraphism. Limb lengths should be measured to rule out limb length inequality. Sitting and standing height should also be measured. Any abnormality indicative of an associated neurologic condition should be further investigated by a neurologist, and further diagnostic studies—such as magnetic resonance imaging of the spinal cord, electromyography, and nerve conduction velocities. When historical or physical findings suggest a diagnosis other than "idiopathic," these studies may assist in making an etiologic diagnosis. Abnormalities detected may also suggest a syndrome requiring genetic consultation.

Spinal deformity is indicated by the presence of body asymmetry (Fig. 1).

TABLE 1. *(Continued).*

Osteochondrodystrophies	Postural	Postexcision (e.g. tumor)
Achondroplasia	Secondary to short leg	Postradiation
Spondyloepiphyseal dysplasia	Due to muscle spasm	Metabolic
Diastrophic dwarfism	Other	Osteoporosis
Mucopolysaccharidoses		Senile
Other	KYPHOSIS	Juvenile
Tumor	Postural	Osteogenesis imperfecta
Benign	Scheuermann disease	Other
Malignant	Congenital	Developmental
Rheumatoid disease	Defect of segmentation	Achondroplasia
Metabolic	Defect of formation	Mucopolysaccharidoses
Rickets	Mixed	Other
Juvenile osteosporosis	Paralytic	Tumor
Osteogenesis imperfecta	Poliomyelitis	Benign
Related to lumbosacral area	Anterior horn cell	Malignant
Spondylolysis	Upper motor neuron	Primary
Spondylolisthesis	Myelomeningocele	Metastatic
Other	Posttraumatic	
Thoracogenic	Acute	LORDOSIS
Postthoracoplasty	Chronic	Postural
Postthoracotomy	Inflammatory	Congenital
Other	Tuberculosis	Paralytic
Hysterical	Other infections	Neuropathic
Functional	Ankylosing spondylitis	Myopathic
	Postsurgical	Contracture of hip flexors
	Postlaminectomy	Secondary to shunts

From Winter (1983), with permission.

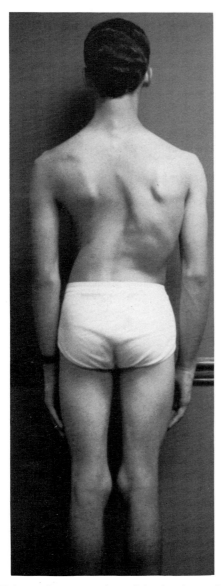

FIG. 1. Asymmetries of the back can be noted in this 15-yr-old boy, distinguished by elevation of the left shoulder area, lateral trunk shift to the right, and prominence of the right-sided rib hump. (From McCarthy (1994).)

The patient should be examined from the front and back, looking for asymmetry in shoulder height, waistline, chest, scapular height, and back prominence. The relation of the thorax to pelvis is noted. Spinal compensation can be measured by dropping a plumb line from the spinous process of C-7 and measuring the distance it falls from the midgluteal cleft.

Rotational asymmetry is best seen by the Adams forward bend test (Fig. 2). Any leg length inequality should be compensated for by placing an appropriate-sized block underneath the short leg. The test is performed by having the patient stand with the feet together and the knees straight. The patient bends forward at the waist with the arms dependent and the hands held with palms opposed (Fig. 3). The rotational asymmetry is best assessed by viewing the patient from in front. The patient should also be viewed from the side to assess any abnormal increases in thoracic or thoracolumbar kyphosis and any evidence of failure to reverse the normal lumbar lordosis.

If on physical examination the patient has evidence of a scoliosis, a standing posteroanterior (PA), unshielded upright radiograph of the spine is ordered. The entire spine, as well as iliac crests, must be included on the radiograph so that no curve is missed and skeletal maturity can be assessed by viewing the ossification of the iliac apophyses (Risser sign). If the patient has complaints of pains or signs of a sagittal spinal deformity, a standing, full-length lateral radiograph of the spine is also ordered to look for conditions such as Scheuermann

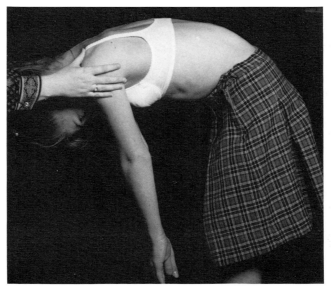

FIG. 2. Adams' forward bend test for school screening. (From McCarthy (1994).)

kyphosis, spondylolysis, or spondy-lolisthesis.

The radiographs are assessed for any congenital abnormalities in the vertebral bodies, ribs, and pelvis. All curves are measured for magnitude (Cobb measurements) and described by direction (direction of the curve convexity), location (e.g., thoracic, lumbar, thoracolumbar, double major, double thoracic), and pedicle rotation (Fig. 4). Maturity is assessed by the Risser sign (Fig. 5). Additional diagnostic and radiographic studies may be indicated if other than idiopathic scoliosis is suspected.

The natural history of a specific curve depends on its cause, pattern, magnitude, and associated sagittal plane deformity. This natural history should be considered in relation to the patient's growth potential as determined by history, phys-ical assessment of maturity, and radiographic assessment of maturity (i.e., Risser sign, ossification of vertebral apophyses, wrist film for bone age assessment, or a combination of these tests).

SCOLIOSIS

Scoliosis is a descriptive term that refers to a lateral curvature of the spine. The scoliosis may be structural or nonstructural. A nonstructural scoliosis corrects or overcorrects on supine side-bending radiographs or traction films. Examples of nonstructural curvatures include scoliosis secondary to limb length inequality or scoliosis secondary to a herniated nucleus pulposus with nerve root irritation causing a list. If the primary problem is corrected (e.g., nerve root irritation), the scoliosis usually resolves. A

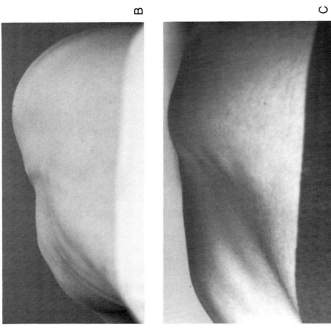

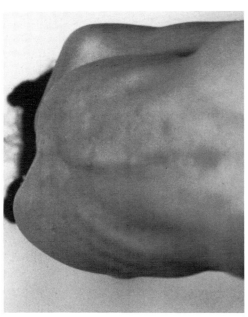

FIG. 3. The forward bend test gives the best visualization of truncal asymmetries in different areas of the spine depending upon the degree of forward extension. **A:** The high thoracic spine. **B:** The midthoracic spine. **C:** The lumbar spine. (From McCarthy (1994).)

structural scoliosis is a fixed lateral curvature with rotation. On radiograph, the spinous processes in a structural curve rotate to the curve concavity. On a supine side-bending radiograph or a traction radiograph, a structural curve lacks normal flexibility. Many conditions are associated with structural scoliosis (see Table 1). The most common structural curvature has no known cause and is referred to as *idiopathic scoliosis*. Though many etiologic theories have been proposed, the cause remains unknown.

Idiopathic scoliosis is usually subclassified into three groups by age at onset of the condition: infantile (0 to 3 yr of age), juvenile (3 to 10 yr of age), and adolescent (older than 10 yr of age but before maturity). Although these subtypes may represent a continuum of the same condition, their natural histories differ. Therefore, these three subtypes of idiopathic scoliosis are considered separately.

Infantile-Onset Idiopathic Scoliosis

Infantile-onset idiopathic scoliosis accounts for less than 1% of all cases of idiopathic scoliosis in the United States. Most of these curves develop within the first 6 mo of life, with the left lumbar curve pattern being the most common. Epidemiologic and associated problems include older maternal age, increased incidence of inguinal hernias among relatives, congenital heart disease (2.5%), congenital hip dysplasia (3.5%), and developmental problems, particularly mental retardation (13%). Of these patients 83% have plagiocephaly, and more than half have evidence of rib-molding deformities, which has led some to theorize intrauterine molding as an etiologic agent. Of the curves 85% regress spontaneously, particularly if the curve onset was before 12 mo of age. The other 15% often progress to severe deformities. Compensatory curves are generally not seen in patients with infantile idiopathic scoliosis. The development of a compensatory curve is a bad prognostic sign that indicates a probable curve progression.

The differential diagnosis in this age group (0 to 3 yr) includes congenital scoliosis and scoliosis of a neuromuscular etiology or intraspinal pathology (e.g., syringomyelia). As this condition is so unusual in North America, MRI of the brain and spinal cord is probably indicated if a careful neurologic exam and evaluation by a pediatric neurologist is negative. The MRI will determine if there is any intraspinal, brain, or cord lesion resulting in the curvature.

If the patient can sit or stand, upright PA and lateral radiographs should be obtained. The Cobb angle and the rib-vertebral angle difference should be measured (Fig. 6). If the rib-vertebral angle difference is greater than 20°, the curvature will probably be progressive. With measurements of less than 20°, the curve is likely to resolve. All patients should be followed by serial radiographic examination, calculating the Cobb angle and the rib-vertebral angle difference at each visit. In progressive curves, the convex side rib head is overlapped by the shadow of the vertebral body. This radiographic sign indicates a progressive curve. Curves that maintain a Cobb angle of less than 35° have a high likelihood of resolution.

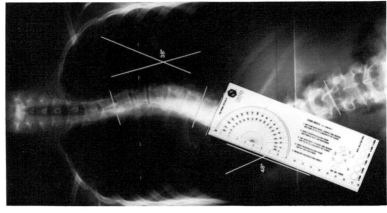

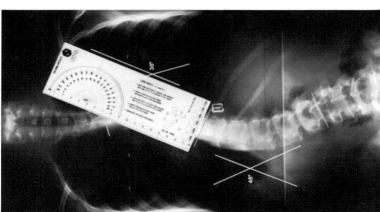

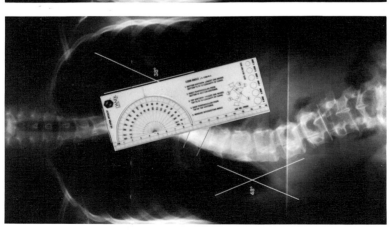

A, B

C

FIG. 4. Cobb method for scoliosis measurement using transparent ruler. Lines are drawn across the top of the vertebral body that best represents the curve and the bottom of the lowest vertebral body in the curve; perpendiculars to these lines intersect, and that angle is the Cobb angle. **A** and **B** show measurement of the thoracic curve.

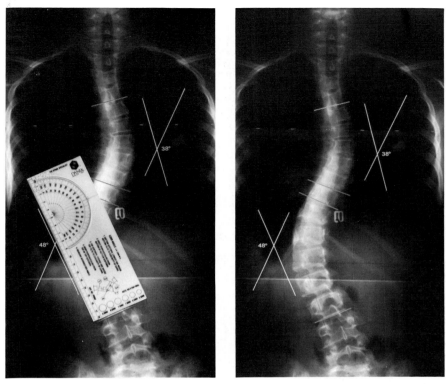

FIG. 4. *(Continued).* **C** and **D** show measurement of the lumbar curve. **E** shows completed curve measurements. (From McCarthy (1994).)

Curves with less than a 25° Cobb angle and less than a 20° rib-vertebral angle difference should be observed, with the patient being re-evaluated in 4 to 6 mo with repeat radiographs. With resolution of the curvature, the patient can be followed at 1- to 2-yr intervals. In curves with a 25° to 35° Cobb angle and with a rib-vertebral angle difference of 25°, repeat clinical and radiographic evaluation at 4- to 6-mo intervals is warranted. If the Cobb angle increases by 5° to 10° with or without changes in the rib-vertebral angle difference, treatment is indicated.

Initial treatment for a progressive curve is serial casting to correct the deformity followed by the use of a Milwaukee brace to maintain correction. In the infantile patient, the corrective cast usually needs to be applied with sedation or under general anesthesia. The casts are worn for 6 to 12 wk and are serially changed until maximum correction is obtained. A Milwaukee brace is then fabricated and worn full-time (22 to 23 hr per day) for 2 to 3 yr to maintain the correction obtained by casting. If the correction is maintained, the patient may be gradually weaned from the brace. If progression occurs, full-time orthotic use must be reinstituted. With rapid curve progression or progression despite brac-

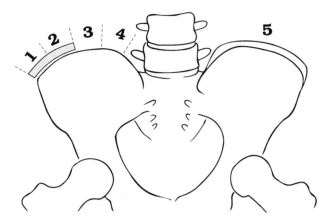

FIG. 5. Risser sign. The Risser sign is a reflection of skeletal maturity. Risser 1, initial appearance of lateral ossification of iliac apophysis; Risser 2, migration halfway across the top of the iliac wing; Risser 3, three fourths of the distance; Risser 4, ossification crossing the iliac wing; Risser 5, complete ossification of the iliac apophysis. (From McCarthy (1994).)

ing, complete neurologic evaluation and MRI should be repeated.

If curve progression continues despite the use of an orthotic, posterior subcutaneous distraction spinal instrumentation without fusion and possible anterior vertebral apical arrest followed by bracing are indicated. The rod can then be lengthened periodically to allow for growth with a formal posterior spinal fusion and instrumentation at maturity.

Juvenile-Onset Idiopathic Scoliosis

Patients classified as having juvenile idiopathic scoliosis may actually have

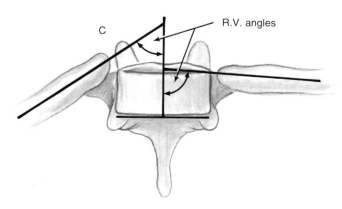

FIG. 6. Measurement of Mehta's rib-vertebra angles. (From Warner (1994).)

late-onset infantile idiopathic scoliosis or early-onset adolescent idiopathic scoliosis. This group of patients accounts for about 20% of all patients with idiopathic scoliosis. These patients, like those with infantile onset, must have a careful neurologic exam and also should have an MRI to rule out brain or intraspinal abnormality. Juvenile-onset idiopathic scoliosis occurs more commonly in girls, with right thoracic curves accounting for two thirds of all curve patterns. Double major curves (right thoracic and left lumbar) and thoracolumbar curves follow in frequency.

Juvenile-onset adolescent idiopathic curvatures may cause severe deformity. Some progress relentlessly from onset, but others progress slowly until the adolescent growth spurt when rapid progression ensues. Unlike infantile curves, juvenile idiopathic scoliosis curvatures do not resolve spontaneously.

Treatment is indicated for a progressive curve of 25° or more. The rib-vertebral angle difference has not been shown to be prognostic in these patients. Curves rarely progress more than 1° per mo. Therefore, if the patient has a curve of less than 20°, follow-up evaluation in 6 to 8 mo is appropriate. Treatment is indicated for progression of at least 10°.

Curves between 20° and 25° at detection should be followed clinically and radiographically in 5 to 6 mo, with treatment indicated for a greater than 5° increase in curve. For curves greater than 25°, because of the high probability of progression, treatment should begin immediately.

If the curve is flexible, as determined by clinical evaluation and in some cases by supine side-bending radiographs, orthotic treatment is indicated in an attempt to prevent further progression. If the curve is rigid, serial cast correction, much like that recommended for infantile idiopathic scoliosis, should be done before fitting the patient with a Milwaukee brace. The orthosis is worn full-time for several years until curve correction is achieved. Then, weaning may begin and continue as long as curve correction is maintained. The brace is then worn at night only until the patient reaches skeletal maturity (i.e., Risser Grade 4 or 5 or no spinal growth for the previous 18 mo).

If the curve progresses rapidly or cannot be controlled by casting or an orthosis, neurologic re-evaluation and possibly MRI (looking for brain and intraspinal lesions) should be considered. If curve progression continues despite casting or bracing, posterior distraction instrumentation without fusion and possible anterior apical arrest should be considered (Fig. 7). After surgery, the patient continues in an orthosis. The distraction device is lengthened with growth until the patient reaches puberty, when posterior spinal fusion and instrumentation are performed.

Adolescent-Onset Idiopathic Scoliosis

Adolescent-onset idiopathic scoliosis accounts for about 80% of cases of idiopathic scoliosis. This condition affects 2% to 3% of the at-risk population (10- to 16-yr-olds). The prevalence in boys and girls is equal in small curves (10°). With increasing curve magnitude (curves greater than 30°), there is an overwhelming female predominance (10:1).

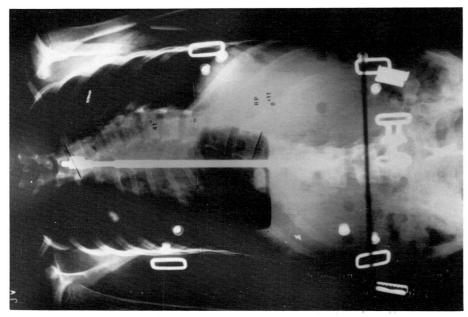

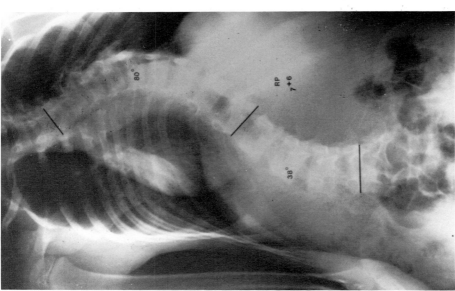

FIG. 7. A: Male aged 7 yr 6 mo with an 80° curve. **B:** One year and 5 mo after insertion of a Moe subcutaneous rod with fusion at hook sites.

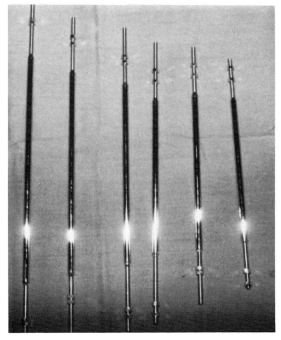

C

FIG. 7. *(Continued).* **C:** Moe subcutaneous rods.

Four major curve patterns are seen in adolescent idiopathic scoliosis (Fig. 8). Because most thoracic curve patterns are convex to the right, a child presenting with a left convex thoracic curve should raise a heightened index of suspicion of underlying pathology. These children should be examined carefully for a neurologic deficit. In this situation, neurologic consultation and MRI scanning is considered a necessity because of the high association of intraspinal abnormality with this curve pattern. Also, a history of rapid progression of an adolescent curvature should alert the physician to consider similar diagnostic evaluations.

Initial radiographic evaluation includes PA and lateral radiographs of the entire spine taken with the patient in the standing position. At follow-up visits, only PA radiographs are usually necessary. It is important to minimize the radiation exposure. Radiation protection measures include beam collimation, antiscatter grids, beam filtration, high-speed film, intensifying screens, gonadal and breast shields, and PA as opposed to anteroposterior (AP) projections. The use of PA projection avoids radiation to the developing breast tissue, which is radiosensitive. Special radiographic views, such as side-bending radiographs, are rarely indicated unless the patient is being considered for surgical management. Each radiograph is measured for the Cobb angle, rotation, and ossification of the iliac apophysis (Risser sign).

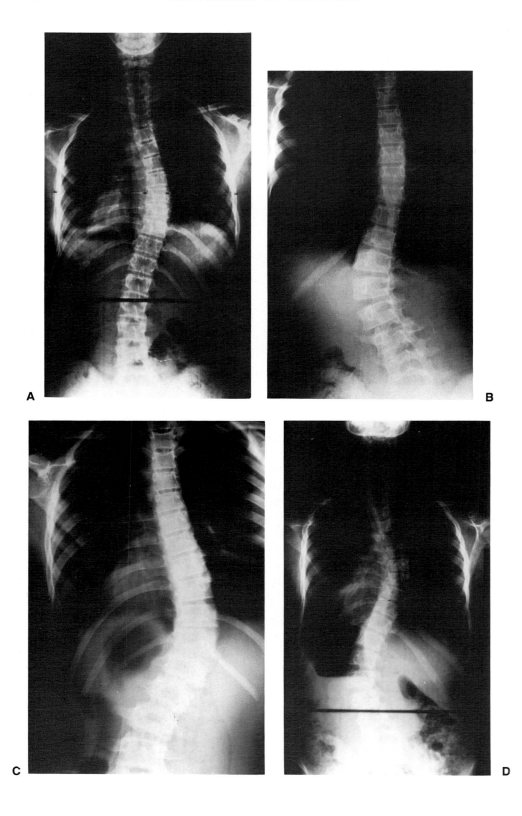

Most treatment decisions are based on curve progression or the probability of curve progression. The factors that influence the probability of curve progression in the immature patient include growth potential factor (age, gender, and maturity) and curve factors (type and magnitude). Double-curved patterns have a greater tendency for progression than do single-curve patterns. Curves detected before menarche have a much greater chance of progression than do those detected after menarche. With increasing age at detection, there is a decreasing risk of curve progression. The larger the curve magnitude at detection, the greater the chance of progression; the lower the Risser grade at curve detection, the greater the risk of progression. The risk of progression in boys is less than that of girls with comparable curves.

The risk of curve progression decreases with increasing skeletal maturity. Large-magnitude curves, however, may continue to progress after maturity (Table 2). In general, curves less than 30° at maturity tend not to progress regardless of the curve pattern. Many curves greater than 30°, and particularly thoracic curves greater than 50°, continue to progress throughout life.

TABLE 2. *Probabilities of progression based on curve magnitude and age*

Curve magnitude at detection (degrees)	Age		
	10–12 yr	13–15 yr	16 yr
<19	25%	10%	0%
20–29	60%	40%	10%
30–59	90%	70%	30%
>60	100%	90%	70%

The incidence of back pain in scoliosis patients is comparable to that in the general population (60% to 80%). Scoliosis patients, however, often have increased frequency of back pain. Patients with lumbar and thoracolumbar curves, particularly those with lateral listhesis or translatory shifts (Fig. 9) at the lower end of their curves, tend to have a greater incidence of backache than do patients with other curve patterns. Back pain in adult patients with scoliosis is not always related to the primary curvature; it may be discogenic, neurogenic, or facet joint related.

Only with thoracic curves is there a direct correlation between decreasing vital capacity and forced expiratory volume (FEV), with increasing curve severity. In all other curve patterns in idiopathic scoliosis, there is no direct correlation between curve magnitude and limitation

FIG. 8. A: Thoracic curve. Ninety percent right convexity involving an average of six vertebrae: apex T-8, T-9; upper end vertebrae T-5, T-6; lower end vertebrae T-11, T-12. **B:** Lumbar curve. Seventy percent left convexity involving an average of five vertebrae: apex L-1, L-2; upper end vertebrae T-11, T-12; lower end vertebrae L-3, L-4. **C:** Thoracolumbar curve. Eighty percent right convexity involving an average of six to eight vertebrae: apex T-11, T-12; upper end vertebrae T-6, T-7; lower end vertebrae L-1, L-2. **D:** Double curve. Ninety percent right thoracic convexity and left lumbar convexity. Thoracic component averages five vertebrae: apex T-7, upper end vertebrae T-5, T-6; lower end vertebra T-10. Lumbar component averages five vertebrae: apex L-2, upper end vertebrae T-11; lower end vertebra L-4. (From Weinstein (1994).)

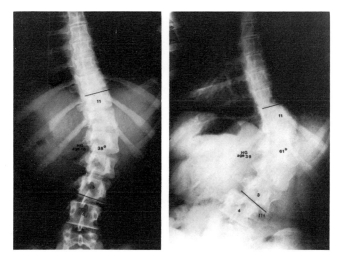

FIG. 9. Sixteen-year-old girl with 38° right lumbar curve from T-11 to L-3 (*left*). Her skeletal maturity is assessed as Grade 5 on the Risser scale. At age 39, her right lumbar curve has increased to 61° (*right*). Note the translatory shift of L-3 on L-4 (*arrows*). (From Weinstein (1994).)

in pulmonary function. Loss of thoracic kyphosis (hypokyphosis), often associated with idiopathic scoliosis, can further diminish pulmonary function associated with increasing curve severity.

Patients do not die from adolescent-onset idiopathic scoliosis. The only patients at risk are those with high-angled (greater than 100°) thoracic curvatures. In these patients, mortality rates are significantly increased because of secondary cor pulmonale and right ventricular failure.

Scoliosis has no adverse effects on pregnancy. The reproductive experiences of women with scoliosis are the same as those of nonscoliotic women. Whether pregnancy causes curve progression is unknown, with evidence on both sides of the issue.

Few patients with adolescent idiopathic scoliosis ever require active treatment (less than 10%). It is important to indi-

vidualize all treatment decisions, taking into consideration the probabilities of progression based on the curve magnitude, skeletal and sexual maturity of the patient, and age of the patient. The general indications for treatment are a progressive curve of 25° or more in a skeletally immature patient. In a skeletally immature patient with a curve of less than 19°, curve progression of at least 10° should be documented before instituting treatment. If the curve is between 20° and 29°, progression of at least 5° should be documented before instituting treatment. If a curve on initial evaluation is over 30°, because of the high probability (over 90%) of progression, no documentation of progression is necessary, and treatment should be initiated immediately. Because curves rarely progress at more than 1° per mo and because the measurement error in scoliosis films is between 3° and 7°, follow-up appointments can be scheduled accordingly.

The standard of nonsurgical treatment for adolescent idiopathic scoliosis has been the Milwaukee brace. Despite widespread use, few long-term studies have evaluated the results of treatment with the Milwaukee brace. In most of the studies performed, curve progression was not documented; thus, it is uncertain whether the scoliosis of those patients braced would have continued to progress had they not been braced.

Reviews of the few retrospective studies that are available show that bracing seems to alter the natural history of curve progression. The purpose of bracing is to stop curve progression. It is generally accepted that the curve progression can be arrested in 85% to 90% of at-risk patients. The most common response to bracing is a moderate amount of correction while the brace is worn, with slow, steady progression of the curve back to the original magnitude after weaning from the brace. Occasionally, maintenance of correction obtained in the brace occurs in some patients who achieve at least 50% reduction in their curvature during the course of treatment. The brace is worn 22 to 23 hr a day and is removed only for bathing or sporting activities. When the patient reaches skeletal maturity (i.e., Risser Grade 4 or no spinal growth over an 18-mo period), the patient is gradually weaned out of the brace. The brace is used on a part-time basis followed by nighttime use only so long as no increases in curvature are noted. Bracing is generally thought to be ineffective in patients with curves greater than 40°.

Although full-time bracing has been the standard, many physicians are choosing part-time bracing programs during the day and/or some nighttime-only programs and using underarm orthoses for better compliance. An underarm brace (thoracic-lumbar-sacral orthoses) is generally acceptable for use in curves with an apex of T-8 or below. Electrical stimulation has been shown to be ineffective.

Surgical treatment is indicated if the patient has evidence of curve progression despite bracing or has a curve magnitude that would be unsuccessfully treated by a brace (i.e., greater than 45° to 50° and skeletally immature). In the adult patient with adolescent idiopathic scoliosis, indications for surgical treatment include pain unresponsive to nonsurgical treatment and documented curve progression.

Surgical treatment of adolescent idiopathic scoliosis involves a posterior spinal fusion in combination with one of the various forms of spinal instrumentation. The purpose of the procedure is to obtain a spinal fusion. Instrumentation is used to correct the deformity and prevent bending of the fusion mass. The standard surgical procedure for the treatment of adolescent idiopathic scoliosis is spinal fusion in conjunction with a Harrington spinal distraction rod. The Harrington rod is used in combination with various other implants and fixation devices. Over the past decade, the use of Harrington rods has been supplanted by various posterior derotation systems (Cotrell Dubousset, TSR, ISOLA, etc.) introduced for correction of the coronal and sagittal plane deformities.

CONGENITAL SPINAL DEFORMITY

Congenital spinal deformities are due to abnormalities of vertebral development. These may result in scoliosis, kyphosis, lordosis, or combinations thereof. Deformities may be of three structural types: failure of formation (e.g., hemivertebrae); failure of segmentation (e.g., unilateral unsegmented bar); or combinations of defects of segmentation and formation (Fig. 10). The resultant deformity is related to the location and type of the congenital anomaly and to the growth potential of the unaffected segments; for example, a lateral segmentation defect causes a pure scoliosis, a posterolateral segmentation defect causes a lordoscoliosis, and an anterior failure of segmentation causes a kyphosis. With defects of formation, any portion of the vertebrae may be hypoplastic or absent. Absence of a vertebral body causes a pure kyphosis, and presence of the posterolateral portion of the vertebrae causes a kyphoscoliosis. Spina bifida results from failure of formation of various portions of the posterior elements.

Patients with congenital scoliosis may have other associated congenital abnormalities. The most frequently affected

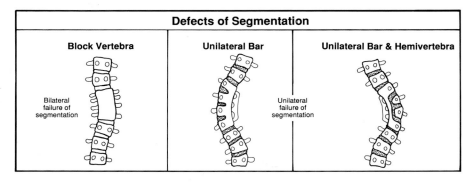

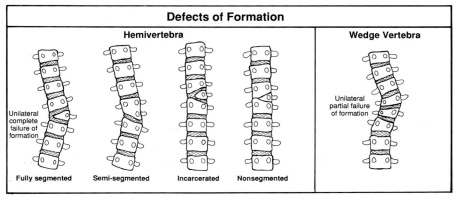

FIG. 10. Congenital scoliosis. (From McMaster (1994).)

systems are the genitourinary, cardiac, and spinal cord. Most congenital spine deformities are discovered only incidentally on radiographs taken for other reasons. Isolated congenital vertebral abnormalities are not thought to have genetic implications.

Severe functional and cosmetic deformities may result from progressive, untreated congenital spinal anomalies. Spinal cord compression and paralysis may occur from a congenital deformity with a kyphotic component. Early detection and careful follow-up of these patients is imperative.

Up to 20% of patients have associated spinal dysraphism (e.g., tethered cord, diastematomyelia, dural lipoma); they must therefore have a careful and detailed neurologic examination. Subtle findings, such as limb atrophy or mild foot abnormalities, may be the only evidence of spinal dysraphism. The skin over the spine should be inspected for hair patches, dimpling, cyst formation, and hemangiomas, which are often associated with a spinal dysrhaphic condition. The chest wall should be examined for any evidence of defects or asymmetry.

About 15% of patients with congenital scoliosis have associated cardiac abnormalities. Any cardiac abnormality detected should be evaluated by a cardiologist.

Twenty percent of patients with congenital spinal abnormalities have an associated abnormality in the genitourinary tract. Six percent of these genitourinary tract abnormalities are potentially life threatening. Renal ultrasound is generally sufficient to provide a screening test for genitourinary tract abnormalities. Evaluation of the lower tracts, however,

may require an intravenous pyelogram (IVP) or retrograde urograms. The kidneys can be seen well on the MRI.

In infancy, supine AP and lateral radiographs are best to evaluate spinal abnormalities. These films provide the best detail of the congenital abnormalities (Fig. 11). A baseline lateral radiograph should be obtained to assess any associated lordosis or kyphosis. Sagittal plane deformity may progress without progression of the scoliosis. Follow-up radiographs can be taken in the standing position (when possible) and measured by the Cobb angle to follow the curve progression.

Each radiograph should be evaluated for gross abnormalities, such as hemivertebrae or nonsegmented vertebrae. The ribs should be examined for congenital abnormalities, and all pedicles should be counted, disc spaces examined, and growth potential assessed. The prognosis for congenital deformities depends on the presence of asymmetric growth. Pedicular widening may be a sign of diastematomyelia, especially in patients with cutaneous or clinical manifestations of spinal dysraphism. Polytomography may be helpful in defining some congenital lesions, particularly in older patients. MRI is indicated if the patient has any evidence of spinal dysraphism. Patients with severe scoliosis may require myelographic enhanced computed tomographic scanning to better define any intraspinal pathology.

In general, about half of all congenital spine anomalies have significant enough progression to require treatment. The natural history of congenital spinal deformities relates specifically to the location of the abnormality, the type of abnor-

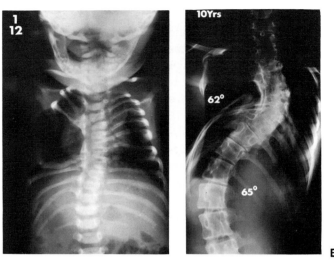

FIG. 11. A: An infant aged 1 mo who had a radiograph because of asymmetry of the thoracic cage. This showed that the spine was relatively straight, but there were absent ribs and a unilateral unsegmented bar extending from T-3 to T-7 on the left. No treatment was given. **B:** By the age of 10 yr, the unilateral unsegmented bar had produced a 62° right upper thoracic scoliosis. However, the main deformity was caused by the secondary development of a severe left structural thoracolumbar scoliosis, which contained no congenital anomalies. (From McMaster (1994).)

mality, and the patient's spinal growth potential. By counting the number of growth centers, as represented by the pedicles on the concave and convex sides of the curve, as well as examining the quality of the disc spaces between vertebrae, an estimate of the probability of curve progression can be made. If there is greater growth potential in the convexity of the curve than the concavity, progression is certain. The worst prognosis for progression of congenital anomalies is the unilateral unsegmented bar opposite to a convex hemivertabrae; this is followed by the unilateral unsegmented bar and the double-convex hemivertebrae (Fig. 11).

The younger the patient at the age of detection, the more likely the patient is to have a progressive deformity. If a con-

genital anomaly is detected at an older age or only incidentally, it rarely causes significant problems. The prognosis for progression in patients with hemivertebrae is difficult to predict in that there are three types of hemivertebrae: fully segmented (worst prognosis), semisegmented, and nonsegmented (most benign).

Stable, nonprogressive curves require only observation until skeletal maturity. Patients with congenital spinal deformity should be followed with radiographs every 6 mo during the first 3 yr of life. If the curve remains stable, follow-up can be on a yearly basis until the adolescent growth spurt, when repeat evaluations every 6 mo may be warranted.

Congenital spinal deformities tend to be rigid; therefore, bracing is generally not a treatment option. The Milwaukee brace, however, can be used in certain situations, particularly in long, flexible curves or compensatory curves above or below congenital abnormalities.

Surgical stabilization is indicated for curve progression regardless of age. In certain instances in which the natural history is well known (e.g., unilateral unsegmented bar opposite a convex hemivertebrae), surgical stabilization is indicated without documentation of progression. Posterior spinal fusion without instrumentation is the standard method of surgical stabilization. The deformity is then corrected by a plaster cast. This type of treatment is at times (particularly in the young patient) associated with bending of the fusion mass. Promising results have been reported with combination anterior hemiepiphysiodesis and posterior hemiarthrodesis, even demonstrating correction for some curves by growth on the unfused concave side.

Distraction instrumentation may be used in certain cases but is associated with an increased risk of neurologic deficit. If correction of the congenital spinal deformity is contemplated, thorough investigation for intraspinal pathology (e.g., MRI or contrast-enhanced CT scanning) must be done prior to surgery. The presence of a diastematomyelia without neurologic deficit does not require treatment. If correction of the spinal deformity is contemplated, however, the diastematomyelia must be addressed surgically. Hemivertebrae excision may be considered in cases of a lumbosacral hemivertebrae with spinal decompensation.

Treatment of congenital kyphotic deformities is surgical. Patients with failure of formation causing either pure kyphosis or kyphoscoliosis are at high risk for spinal cord compression. Posterior hemivertebrae or failure of formation of a vertebral body should be treated by immediate surgical stabilization. These patients generally benefit from a combined anteroposterior surgical spinal fusion.

With failures of segmentation, a progressive kyphosis may ensue, although this rarely leads to neurologic deficit. A short, posterior fusion arrests spinal growth and halts progression of the deformity. If the deformity exceeds 50°, anterior fusion must be done in conjunction with the posterior spinal fusion; otherwise progression may occur by bending of the fusion mass. Any neurologic deficit associated with congenital kyphosis or congenital kyphoscoliosis must be treated by spinal cord decompression and stabilization.

CONDITIONS ASSOCIATED WITH BACK PAIN

In contrast to adults, back pain in children is not a common complaint. It must therefore be carefully evaluated. The normal child may have occasional complaints of back pain after strenuous physical activity, prolonged sitting or standing, or repetitive heavy lifting. Back pain may also accompany a viral illness. Repetitive or chronic backache symptoms should be carefully investigated. There are many causes of backache in children (Table 3), and the cause can be established in about 85% of cases.

The child and family should be questioned to quantitate and characterize the pain. The pain should be characterized

TABLE 3. *Causes of back pain in children*

Tumors
  Spine
  Spinal cord
Herniated nucleus pulposus
Spondylolysis
Spondylolisthesis
Scheuermann kyphosis
Postural kyphosis
Vertebral osteomyelitis
Discitis
Overuse syndromes
Rheumatologic condition

as to nature, intensity, location, and time of occurrence. By taking a careful history, the physician should be able to narrow the possible sources of the back pain. For example, if the patient is complaining of back pain usually at night with symptoms relieved by aspirin, an osteoid osteoma or osteoblastoma should be suspected. Pain during athletic events, such as gymnastics or blocking in a football lineman, are suggestive of spondylolysis or spondylolisthesis. Leg pain with or without associated back pain may be radicular pain associated with a herniated nucleus pulposus or may be secondary to hamstring tightness because of cauda equina irritation from a spondylolysis or spondylolisthesis. Back pain in children with or without neurologic deficits may also be a manifestation of intraspinal abnormalities.

Physical examination of the child presenting with the chief complaint of back pain should consist of a general overall evaluation, including examination of the head and neck, the upper and lower extremities, gait, and spine. A careful, detailed neurologic examination, includ-

ing muscle, reflex, and sensory testing, is mandatory. Any loss of normal spine motion or failure to reverse lumbar lordosis on forward flexion is suggestive of a pathologic condition and should be investigated.

The back should be palpated for any areas of tenderness over the spine or paraspinous region. The flank should be percussed, looking for areas of tenderness that may indicate a visceral abnormality. The abdomen should be palpated for masses. Limb lengths should be measured. Thighs and calves should be measured for any evidence of atrophy. Straight leg raising tests are performed looking for signs of nerve root irritation or excessive hamstring tightness. The sacroiliac region, particularly the sacroiliac joints, should be examined for any signs of joint pathology. Signs of meningeal irritation should be sought.

Supine AP and lateral radiographs of the involved area of the spine are taken to assess bony detail. Standing PA and lateral radiographs can be ordered if the patient is being assessed for scoliosis or kyphosis associated with the pain. If spondylolisthesis or spondylolysis is suspected, a cone-down lateral view of the L3-S1 region should be ordered. Oblique views may also be helpful.

If plain films are negative, special studies may be warranted. Bone scanning is useful in the face of a negative radiograph in diagnosing stress fractures, bone tumors, or infections of the spine. CT scanning may be helpful in documenting the anatomic details of lesions seen on plain films. For soft tissue lesions around the spine or for evaluating the spinal cord, MRI is the diagnostic procedure of choice.

Depending on the patient's clinical history, physical examination, and radiographic findings, certain laboratory studies may be helpful. A complete blood count and an erythrocyte sedimentation rate, although nonspecific, may be abnormal in infections, tumors, or rheumatologic conditions. If a collagen disease is suspected, HLA-B27 and rheumatoid factors may help in the diagnosis.

Scheuermann Kyphosis

Normal thoracic kyphosis is generally accepted to be between 20° and 45°. The degree of kyphosis in the thoracic spine increases with age. Kyphosis should never be present at the thoracolumbar junction. Any kyphotic deformity present at this level is considered abnormal.

Scheuermann kyphosis is a structural sagittal plane deformity in the thoracic or the thoracolumbar spine. Patients have an increased kyphosis in the thoracic or thoracolumbar spine with associated diagnostic radiographic changes. The diagnosis of Scheuermann kyphosis is usually made during the adolescent growth spurt and is rarely found in patients younger than 10 yr. An increased incidence of spondylolysis and spondylolisthesis is reported in patients with Scheuermann kyphosis as well as a 20% to 30% incidence of an associated scoliosis in the region of the kyphosis.

Many theories have been advanced as to the cause of the condition, including mechanical, metabolic, and endocrinologic. There is a definite hereditary component, but no mode of inheritance is known. Patients with Scheuermann kyphosis are generally taller than comparably aged patients, and their skeletal age is advanced over their chronologic age.

The two types of thoracic Scheuermann kyphosis are kyphosis with the apex at the T7-9 level and kyphosis with the apex in the lower thoracic spine at the thoracolumbar junction (T11-12). There is generally an associated secondary increased lumbar lordosis. The so-called lumbar Scheuermann kyphosis has the apex at L1-2. This condition is generally more common in boys and in young athletes. It is thought to have a traumatic cause.

Clinically, most patients with thoracic Scheuermann kyphosis present with a history of deformity. The child is often brought in by the parent because of poor posture or is referred from a school screening program. The incidence of pain in the adolescent is low, although about 20% of patients present with a history of discomfort in the region of the kyphosis. In patients with lumbar Scheuermann kyphosis, the chief complaint is generally pain (80%). The pain is usually intermittent. It is characteristically is dull and aching and is generally activity related and relieved by rest.

On physical examination, patients with upper thoracic Scheuermann disease present with a kyphotic deformity. This is best demonstrated in the forward flexed position (Fig. 12). The flexibility of the kyphosis can be demonstrated by having the patient either hyperextend from a prone position or sit on a chair with the hands held behind the head and hyperextend. Lack of flexibility indicates the structural nature of the kyphotic deformity in contrast to patients with flexible postural kyphosis. Hyperlordosis in the

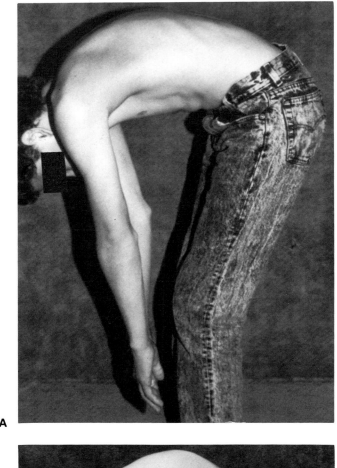

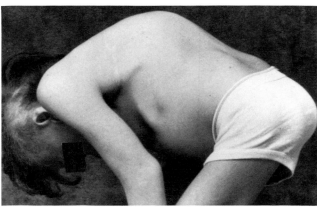

FIG. 12. A: Normal thoracic kyphosis on forward bend test in a 15-yr-old boy. **B:** Congenital kyphosis on forward bend test in an 11-yr-old boy.

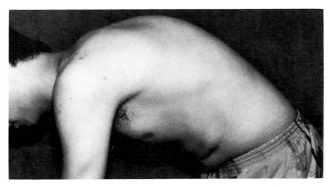

FIG. 12. *(Continued).* **C:** Scheuermann's kyphosis on forward bend test in a 17-yr-old boy. (From McCarthy (1994).)

lumbar spine is also present. In lower thoracic Scheuermann disease, the kyphotic deformity is at the thoracolumbar junction. There may also be hypokyphosis above the thoracolumbar junction and hypolordosis in the lumbar spine.

Because of the high association of scoliosis with Scheuermann kyphosis, this must be assessed. The thoracic Scheuermann patient may have tenderness to palpation above or below the apex of the kyphosis. In the lumbar variety, tenderness to palpation is generally in the region of the curve apex.

Each patient should have a careful neurologic examination. Although rare, at extreme degrees of kyphosis, neurologic deficit can ensue. In addition, there is an association of epidural cyst, causing spastic paraparesis in patients with Scheuermann kyphosis. Hamstring tightness may be present.

Very few data are available regarding the natural history of Scheuermann kyphosis. Many authors think that, in the thoracic variety, if pain is present it subsides with growth and that there are few adverse long-term sequelae of the condition. Others believe that the incidence of pain with Scheuermann kyphosis increases throughout life, as may the deformity. The pain in adults with Scheuermann disease is generally described as a feeling of tiredness in the back. These patients may have pain in the hyperlordotic lumbar spine or at the apex of the kyphosis because of ankylosis.

The diagnosis of Scheuermann kyphosis is confirmed on a standing lateral radiograph of the spine. The radiograph should be taken with the arms parallel to the floor and resting on a support (Fig. 13). It is important to see the entire spine to measure the thoracic kyphosis, lumbar lordosis, and any secondary cervicothoracic curves that may accompany the kyphosis. The kyphosis is measured by determining the angle between the maximally tilted end vertebrae (similar to the Cobb method for measuring scoliosis). A PA scoliosis film should be obtained to detect the presence and magnitude of any associated scoliosis.

Radiographic diagnosis is made by the presence of irregularities of the vertebral endplates, anterior vertebral body wedg-

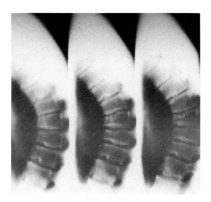

FIG. 13. Typical radiographic alterations of Scheuermann kyphosis with vertebral endplate erosions, vertebral wedging, Schmorl's hernias (nodules), and dorsal hyperkyphosis. (From Ascani and La Rosa (1994).)

ing, Schmorl nodes, and decreased intervertebral disc space height. In older patients, degenerative changes may be evident. The endplate irregularity, Schmorl nodes, and disc space narrowing are often but not always seen. There is some discrepancy in the literature regarding the number of consecutive vertebrae that need be wedged to make the diagnosis of Scheuermann kyphosis. By the Sorenson criterion, there should be wedging of more than 5° in three or more adjacent vertebrae. In other studies, the diagnosis is made by the presence of only one wedged vertebrae of more than 5°. This compounds the problem of determining the natural history.

On the PA radiograph, any evidence of interpedicular widening should be noted because of the association of epidural cysts with Scheuermann kyphosis. Any scoliosis present should be assessed (curves rarely exceed 20°). The flexibility of the kyphosis is best demon- strated in a supine hyperextension lateral view with a "bump" under the apex of the kyphosis. In lumbar Scheuermann disease, irregularities of the vertebral endplates are usually present, as are Schmorl nodes. The intervertebral disc spaces are normal, and there is no evidence of vertebral wedging.

In a patient with an apparent exaggerated kyphosis, the differential diagnosis includes a postural round back. In postural round back, there is a slight increase in the thoracic kyphosis. The kyphosis, however, is flexible, as demonstrated by prone or sitting hyperextension tests. On the standing lateral radiograph, there are no structural changes as noted for Scheuermann kyphosis. The kyphosis in postural kyphosis patients is usually in the range of 45° to 60°. On the supine hyperextension lateral view, the deformity is totally flexible. The question remains of whether a postural kyphosis left untreated may progress and get secondary bony changes resembling Scheuermann disease. Postural kyphosis, if flexible, should be treated by exercising.

Thoracic hyperkyphosis is also seen in patients with various types of skeletal dysplasia, such as spondyloepiphyseal dysplasia congenita and Morquio disease. These conditions can usually be diagnosed by the clinical examination and other radiographic features. Ankylosing spondylitis may present a similar picture, but 97% of these patients are HLA-B27-positive. Kyphosis may also be present in patients who had a laminectomy before skeletal maturity or who had radiation to the spine for a regional tumor. Kyphosis may also be seen with eosinophilic granuloma. Type II congenital kyphosis (failure of segmentation) may be confused with Scheuermann disease. It may be necessary to use polytomography to identify the anterior failure of segmentation seen in this condition to differentiate it from Scheuermann kyphosis.

Lumbar Scheuermann disease generally responds well to nonoperative measures, such as nonsteroidal antiinflammatory agents and temporary activity restriction. There are no adverse long-term sequelae from lumbar Scheuermann disease.

Some authors think that the natural history of thoracic Scheuermann kyphosis is benign and therefore requires no treatment. Others report increasing pain with progression of the deformity. It is uncertain whether treatment prevents any of the consequences that may occur without treatment. Treatment of Scheuermann kyphosis in the skeletally immature patient is recommended in the hope of preventing excessive deformity that may cause pain and cosmetic concerns. Exercises alone are not beneficial. Hyperextension body casts changed at monthly intervals to correct the curvature may be used in the skeletally immature patient with a rigid Scheuermann kyphosis (i.e., less than 10° to 15° of correction on hyperextension lateral radiograph). Once the correction has been obtained, it can then be maintained using a Milwaukee brace. In those patients with a somewhat flexible Scheuermann kyphosis, the Milwaukee brace is the recommended orthosis. In some centers, particularly in Europe, casting alone is used as a treatment. Treatment is usually continued until the patient reaches skeletal maturity. In immature patients, some of the anterior wedging associated with

Scheuermann kyphosis can be corrected. Follow-up studies of patients treated for Scheuermann kyphosis demonstrate increase of the kyphosis over time even after brace treatment. In patients with curves greater than 75° and with pain unresponsive to nonoperative measures, spinal fusion can be considered. Treatment of kyphosis of this magnitude requires anterior and posterior spinal fusion throughout the length of kyphosis. Cord decompression is indicated for the rare patient who has neurologic deficits secondary to epidural cysts or increased kyphotic angulation both of which are uncommon.

Spondylolysis and Spondylolisthesis

Spondylolysis is a descriptive term referring to a defect in the pars interarticularis. The defect may be unilateral or bilateral and may be associated with spondylolisthesis. *Spondylolisthesis* refers to the anterior displacement (translation) of a vertebra with respect to the vertebra caudal to it. This translation may also be accompanied by an angular deformity (kyphosis). These two topics are considered together in that the most common cause of spondylolisthesis in children is spondylolysis.

Spondylolysis occurs most commonly at L5-S1 and less frequently at the L4-5 region. Spondylolytic lesions may occur at other lumbar regions or at multiple levels. Spondylolytic lesions are found in about 5% of the general population. Spondylolysis is an acquired condition. It has not been reported in infants and is rarely present before 5 yr of age. There is an increased incidence of spondylolysis and spondylolisthesis up to the age of 20 yr, after which the incidence remains stable.

Spondylolysis is thought to be an acquired condition secondary to a stress fracture at the pars intraarticularis. Experimental studies showed that extension movements of the spine, particularly in combination with lateral flexion, increase the shear stress at the pars interarticularis. Clinical evidence for this theory includes the high association (four times more than normal) in female gymnasts, football lineman, and soldiers carrying backpacks. This etiologic theory is also supported by a reported higher association in patients with Scheuermann kyphosis with secondary excessive lumbar lordosis. In contrast, spondylolysis has not been seen in patients who have never walked.

Spondylolisthesis is classified into five types (Table 4). It is further classified by the degree of angular and translational displacement. The diagnosis and treatment of the condition depends on the type.

Spondylolysis and spondylolisthesis may be inherited conditions. There is a high association of the condition in family members of affected patients. There

are racial and gender differences, with the lowest incidence in black females and the highest in white males. Most patients with Type I spondylolisthesis have abnormalities at the lumbosacral junction with poor development of the superior aspect of the sacrum and superior sacral facets and with associated sacral spina bifida. Similar congenital changes have also been reported in about one third of patients with Type II spondylolisthesis. Thus, these conditions may be genetic, acquired, or both.

The presenting complaints of patients with spondylolysis and spondylolisthesis are determined primarily by the age of the patient and, in spondylolisthesis, by the type. Although pain is the most common presenting complaint in the adult, it is relatively uncommon in children or the symptom is usually mild. Children most commonly present with gait abnormalities, posture deformity, and hamstring tightness. Back pain is usually localized to the lower back region, with occasional radiation to the buttocks and thighs. Occasional L5 radiculopathies are present, although this is not common in children.

The adult patient with degenerative spondylolisthesis generally is older than 40 yr of age, and women are more commonly affected than men. Pain in degenerative spondylolisthesis is often similar to the pain patterns in patients with a herniated nucleus pulposus (i.e., the patient has pain radiating down the leg and complaints of sciatica). Patients may complain of pain similar to spinal stenosis and have claudication-type symptoms (i.e., pain and cramping in the calves and back brought on by walking and relieved

TABLE 4. *Classification of spondylolisthesis*

Type	Description
I	Dysplastic
IIA	Fracture in pars interarticularis (stress fracture)
IIB	Elongated intact pars interarticularis
IIC	Acute fracture
III	Degenerative
IV	Traumatic (fracture in other than pars interarticularis)
V	Pathologic

by sitting in a flexed spinal posture). In most cases of spondylolysis and spondylolisthesis, pain is precipitated by activity, especially flexion and extension on a repetitive basis, and relieved by rest or lowered activity levels.

Each patient must have a complete physical examination, including detailed neurologic examination. About 80% of children with spondylolisthesis have evidence of hamstring tightness. The cause for this is unknown but it is thought to be instability in the area of the spondylolysis and spondylolisthesis resulting in cauda equina irritation. Hamstring tightness is responsible for the postural abnormalities often seen as the presenting complaint of the patients with spondylolisthesis. Restrictive flexion secondary to the hamstring tightness and the pelvic tilt gives the patient a stiff-legged gait with a short stride length. The pelvis rotates as the child takes a step, and often the child walks on tiptoes with the knees slightly flexed. The hamstring tightness may be so severe in some children that, in performing a straight leg raising test in a supine position, the leg can only be lifted several inches off the table.

The physical findings referable to the back depend on the type and degree of the slip. Patients may present with mild tenderness to palpation in the area of the spondylolysis or spondylolisthesis. In severe grades of slip, a "step-off" may be palpated. There may be an apparent increase in lumbar lordosis with a backward tilting of the pelvis. The patient may present with protrusion of the lower abdomen, and in severe cases of spondylolisthesis, a deep transverse abdominal crease may be noted. A detailed neurologic examination, including deep tendon reflexes, sensory examination, and motor strength, should be performed on each patient with particular attention to any dysesthesia near the sacrum and rectum. A history of bowel or bladder dysfunction may be indicative of cauda equina syndrome.

About one third of patients with symptomatic spondylolisthesis have evidence of scoliosis. The scoliosis most commonly seen in association with symptomatic spondylolisthesis is generally not structural. It is more commonly seen in patients with high-degree slips. The curve is usually in the lumbar region and resolves with the resolution of the symptoms of the spondylolisthesis. Some patients have a characteristic idiopathic scoliosis that is unaffected by the spondylolisthesis or its treatment.

Spondylolisthesis in patients with isthmic spondylolysis may occur any time after the pars fractures. Most slippage occurs during the adolescent growth spurt. Rarely are significant increases in the degree of spondylolisthesis seen after skeletal maturity.

If spondylolysis or spondylolisthesis is clinically suspected, standing PA and standing lateral radiographs of the spine with a cone-down lateral view of L-3 to the sacrum are indicated. In most cases, the pars interarticular defect can be seen on the spot lateral views. The defect is usually at the L5 to S1 level. Defects at the L-4 level are more common in patients who have complete or partial sacralization of the L5 vertebra. If the defect is not visualized on the lateral film and the condition is suspected, an oblique view may be helpful. On this view, the so-called Scotty dog with a broken neck or wearing a collar can be visualized (Fig. 14). In about 20% of patients, the lytic defect is unilateral and may be accompanied by reactive sclerosis in the opposite pedicle, lamina, or both. This situation often presents a difficult diagnostic dilemma in that the sclerotic region can be confused with lesions such as osteoid osteoma and osteoblastoma. If the lesion is not visualized on plain radiograph, technetium bone scanning may be helpful in identifying the lesion. In an acute injury, a positive bone scan may allow for early detection. Bone scanning is also used to assess whether an established lesion has the potential to heal. If the lesion is "cold," there is an established nonunion, and hence immobilization would probably not result in healing of the stress fracture.

In Type I spondylolisthesis, the entire posterior arch slips forward (Fig. 15). There is dysplasia of superior articular facets of the sacrum and inferior articular facets of L5. Type I slips are generally limited to 25% to 30% slippage unless the pars becomes attenuated or fractures, allowing for severe degrees of slippage to occur.

In Type II spondylolisthesis, the spinous process and posterior elements remain behind (Fig. 15). Other changes should be noted, including the shape of the sacrum (i.e., whether it is flattened or dome-shaped) and the amount of wedging of L5. In the adult disc space, narrowing and degenerative changes at the intervertebral disc and posterior elements should be noted. Patients with a more rounded S1 and a more wedged-shaped L5 have a greater risk of progression.

Spondylolisthesis is graded on a scale of 1 to 4 depending on the percentage of anterior translation of L5 on S1, with grade 1 being a 25% slip; grade 2, a 50% slip; grade 3, a 75% slip; and grade 4, a complete slip. The term *spondyloptosis* is used to describe complete displacement of L5 in front of S1. It is important in assessing spondylolisthetic patients to have standing lateral radiographs of the lumbosacral junction because instability is not uncommon, particularly in childhood. Several standard methods of measurements are used to quantitate spondy-

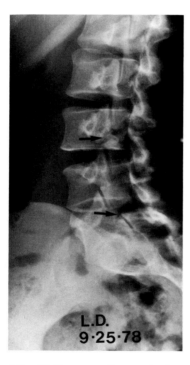

FIG. 14. Oblique radiograph demonstrating pars defects at L-5 and L-3, which correspond to the "collar" on the "Scotty dog." (From Bradford and Hu (1994).)

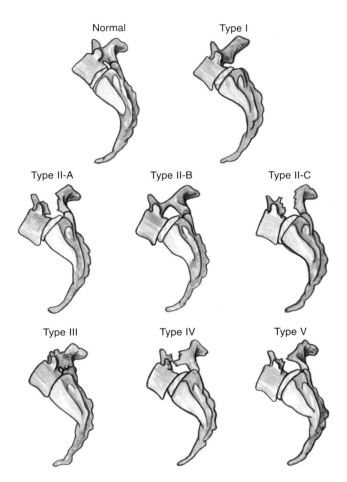

FIG. 15. Classification of spondylolisthesis according to Wiltse. Type I: Dysplastic— Congenital deficiency of the superior sacral and/or inferior fifth lumbar facets with gradual slipping of the fifth lumbar vertebra. Type II: Isthmic—A: Lytic (fatigue fractures of pars); B: Elongated but intact pars; C: Acute fracture. Type III: Degenerative—Degeneration of joints allowing forward displacement, usually L-4 on L-5. Type IV: Traumatic—Acute fracture in areas other than the pars interarticularis. Type V: Pathologic—Attenuation of the pedicle secondary to structural weakness of the bone. Children and adolescents most commonly demonstrate Type I or Type II spondylolisthesis.

lolisthesis; these include the percentage of translation, sagittal roll, and slip angle (Fig. 16). These measurements of angulation or lumbosacral kyphosis are important prognostic indicators.

In the adult patient with degenerative spondylolisthesis additional radiographic studies may be in order. These studies include flexion extension lateral views to detect instability and CT scanning with or without myelographic enhancement to assess the integrity of the disc and to look for other potential sources of the pain. They are also useful to ascertain the specific abnormality in spondylolisthesis associated with or causing spinal stenosis and to rule out intraspinal pathologic conditions in patients who do not have resolution of symptoms by nonoperative measures. Myelography or MRI is rarely indicated in the child or adolescent with spondylolisthesis unless the patient has signs or symptoms of nerve root compression or cauda equina syndrome. In the adult patient, other diagnostic tests, such as EMG, motor nerve condition studies, and psychologic testing, may be considered.

Most children with spondylolysis can be treated successfully without surgery. If the diagnosis is made as an incidental finding, no activity restrictions are necessary. The patient should, however, be followed through skeletal maturity with standing spot lateral radiographs of the lumbosacral spine every 6 mo to watch for the development of spondylolisthesis.

In a patient with spondylolysis with acute onset of symptoms, bone scanning is helpful to assess the lesion and to follow healing. There is some evidence to suggest that immobilization in a cast or brace allows for healing of the lesion in these cases. There are some differences of opinion about whether the cast should extend from the nipple line to include one or both legs or if the same results may be achieved in a thoracic lumbar sacral orthosis (TLSO). If this treatment is attempted, the patient can be followed by serial radiographs and bone scans to assess healing.

Most patients with nonacute lesions can be successfully treated by activity restriction and exercises, including hamstring stretching. If symptoms are more severe, a short period of bed rest may be tried before immobilization in a TLSO. Exercises should be prescribed. Nonsteroidal antiinflammatory medications are a useful adjuvant to treatment.

If conservative management fails, other conditions, including neurologic conditions and tumors of the spine and spinal cord, must be ruled out before instituting surgical treatment. In patients whose symptoms do not respond to nonoperative treatment, lumbosacral intertransverse process fusion of L5 to S1 has a 90% chance of obtaining a solid fusion with relief of symptoms, including resolution of hamstring tightness. In patients with isolated or multiple defects in the L1-4 region, surgical repair of the defect by one of many available techniques is often recommended to allow for sparing of lumbar motion segments.

In asymptomatic patients who have spondylolisthesis with less than a 25% slip, no treatment is indicated. Natural history indicates that the likelihood of having future problems is essentially the same as that of the general population. With slips greater than 25%, there is an

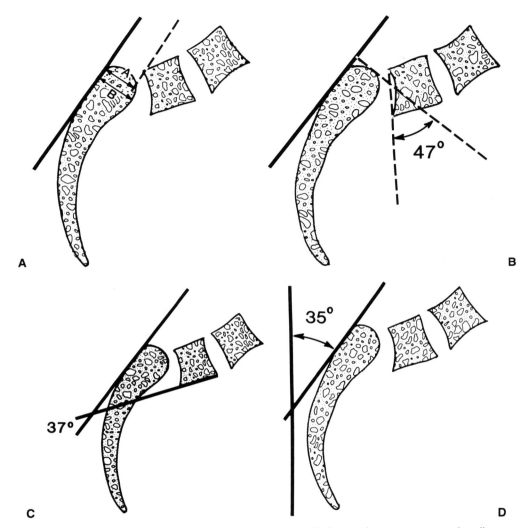

FIG. 16. A: Percentage of slippage is measured relative to the anteroposterior diameter of the sacrum. As shown, A/B x 100 = 72%. **B:** The slippage angle (47° as shown) is determined by drawing a line along the posterior cortex of the sacrum and measuring the angle between its perpendicular and a line drawn along the inferior border of L-5. **C:** Sagittal rotation is the angle measured between the posterior cortex of the sacrum and the anterior cortex of the L-5 vertebral body. **D:** Sacral inclination is the angle between the posterior surface of the sacrum and a vertical line drawn from the floor. Normal sacral inclination is greater than 30°. (From Bradford and Hu (1994).)

increased likelihood of the patient having lower-back symptoms compared with the general population. Certain clinical and radiographic risk factors have been determined to be associated with future pain, progressive deformity, and increasing degree of spondylolisthesis (Table 5).

In the skeletally immature patient with less than a 50% slip, nonoperative measures should be tried in attempt to control symptoms. These measures are similar to those described previously for the treatment of spondylolysis. About two thirds of these patients have resolution of symptoms with nonoperative treatment.

Indications for surgery in the skeletally immature patient are failure of relief of symptoms by nonoperative measures or a slip of greater than 50%. L-4-sacrum intertransverse process fusion is recommended in those patients with a greater than 50% slip, and L5-sacrum fusion is recommended for those patients with a less than 50% slip. Ninety percent of children can expect to have a solid fusion within 1 yr of surgery and gain resolution of any mild neurologic symptoms,

TABLE 5. *Risk factors in spondylolisthesis for pain, progression, and deformity*

CLINICAL RISK FACTORS
Younger age
Female patient
Recurrent symptoms
Hamstring tightness, if associated with gait abnormalities or postural deformity
RADIOGRAPHIC RISK FACTORS
Type I greater risk than Type II
Greater than 50% slip
Increased risk with increased slip angle
L5-S1 instability with rounded sacral dome and vertical sacrum

including hamstring tightness, over the ensuing 12 to 18 mo. Nonunions and curve progression despite a solid fusion, however, have been reported in children undergoing in situ fusion. Because of these problems, particularly with high-grade slips, many authors advocate fusion with closed reduction, followed by pantaloon casting for 3 to 6 mo to decrease the sagittal rotation and improve the cosmetic deformity. Although sagittal role or slip angle can be changed by closed methods, vertebral translation is generally unaltered or is changed little by these techniques. Decompression is rarely necessary in childhood spondylolisthesis and must be accompanied by a fusion to prevent further progression.

In the adult being treated for Type I or Type II spondylolisthesis, associated conditions (e.g., herniated nucleus pulposus) must be ruled out and disc degeneration and nerve compression must be evaluated. In the adult, the symptoms are generally confined to back pain. In situ fusion may be all that is necessary. If the patient has leg pain, decompression and fusion may be warranted. In the adult patient with spondylolisthesis with or without radiculopathy, many surgeons advocate internal fixation along with a spinal fusion. Internal fixation is most commonly attained by means of pedicle screws, plates, or rods. In the adult, because the risk of further displacement is minimal, the pantaloon cast immobilization advocated in children is unnecessary.

In the adult with degenerative spondylolisthesis (Type III), the source of the pain must be sought before recommending surgical treatment. These patients rarely develop spondylolisthesis greater than 25%. Radiographs show evidence of degenerative disc disease as well as degeneration of the facet joints. Some patients develop retrolisthesis, and others may develop intraspinal synovial cysts. A complete diagnostic evaluation must be done including discography to ascertain the source of the pain. Adult patients require a much more extensive work-up, including the possibility of EMG, motor nerve conduction studies, psychologic testing, discography, epidural steroid injections, or nerve root blocks, to ascertain the cause of pain and prognosticate the effectiveness of treatment. Most patients with degenerative spondylolisthesis can also be treated nonoperatively. In those who fail conservative treatment, exhaustive diagnostic measures must be undertaken to determine the source of pain.

Herniated Nucleus Pulposus

Less than 3% of all cases of herniated nucleus pulposus occur in children. An estimated 30% to 60% of cases reported have an associated history of trauma. There is a male predominance. Herniated nucleus pulposus in children is associated with additional vertebral disease, including sacralized L5, lumbarized S1 (either complete or incomplete), asymmetric articular facets, congenital stenosis, and spina bifida.

Symptoms of a herniated nucleus pulposus in the child may be minimal or they may be characteristic of the adult condition. In children, however, there is occasionally an associated scoliosis secondary to muscle spasm. The neurologic symptoms in children are less common and less severe. Herniated nucleus pulposus may also occur in association with a slipped vertebral apophysis or fracture of the vertebral apophysis. The most common levels involved in children are L4-5 and L5-S1. Treatment recommendations are the same as those in the adult.

SUGGESTED READING

1. Ascani E, La Rosa G. Scheuermann's kyphosis. In: Weinstein SL, ed. *The pediatric spine: principles and practice.* New York: Raven Press, 1994; 557–584.
2. Bradford DS, Hu SS. Spondylolysis and spondylolisthesis. In: Weinstein SL, ed. *The pediatric spine: principles and practice.* New York: Raven Press, 1994; 885–601.
3. Bradford DS, Lonstein JE, Moe, JH, Ogilvie JW, Winter RB. *Moe's textbook of scoliosis and spinal deformities.* 2nd ed. Philadelphia: WB Saunders; 1987.
4. Bridwell KH, DeWald RL. *The textbook of spinal surgery.* Philadelphia: JB Lippincott; 1991.
5. Bunnell WA. Back pain in children. *Orthop Clin North Am* 1982;13:587.
6. Fredrickson BE, Baker D, McHolick WJ, et al. The natural history of spondylolysis and spondylolisthesis. *J Bone Joint Surg [Am]* 1984;66A:699.
7. Harris IE, Weinstein SL. Long-term follow-up of patients with Grade III and IV spondylolisthesis: treatment with and without posterior fusion. *J Bone Joint Surg [Am]* 1987; 69A:960.
8. Hensinger RN. Current concepts reviews: spondylolysis and spondylolisthesis in children and adolescents. *J Bone Joint Surg [Am]* 1989;71A:1098.
9. Lonstein JE, Carlson M. Prognostication in idiopathic scoliosis. *J Bone Joint Surg [Am]* 1984;66A:1061.
10. Lonstein JE, Weinstein SL, Keller RB, Englar GL, Tolo VT. AAOS instructional course on adolescent idiopathic scoliosis. *AAOS Instruct Course Lect* 1989;38:105.
11. Lowe TG. Scheuermann's disease and postural round back. *J Bone Joint Surg [Am]* 1990;72A:940.

12. McCarthy RE. Evaluation of the patient with deformity. In: Weinstein SL, ed. *The pediatric spine: principles and practice.* New York: Raven Press, 1994; 185–224.

13. McMaster MJ. Congenital scoliosis. In: Weinstein SL, ed. *The pediatric spine: principles and practice.* New York: Raven Press, 1994; 227–244.

14. McMaster M, David C. Hemivertebrae as a cause of scoliosis: a review of 104 patients. *J Bone Joint Surg [Br]* 1986;68B:588.

15. McMaster M, Ohtsuka K. The natural history of congenital scoliosis: a study of 251 patients. *J Bone Joint Surg [Am]* 1982;64A:1128.

16. Murray PM, Weinstein SL, Spratt K. Natural history and long term follow-up of Scheuermann's kyphosis. *J Bone Joint Surg [Am]* 1993;75A:236–248.

17. Saraste H. Long term clinical and radiographical followup of spondylolysis and spondylolisthesis. *J Pediatr Orthop* 1987;7:631.

18. Warner WC Jr. Juvenile idiopathic scoliosis. In: Weinstein SL, ed. *The pediatric spine: principles and practice.* New York: Raven Press, 1994; 431–444.

19. Weinstein SL. *The pediatric spine: principles and practice.* New York: Raven Press; 1994.

20. Weinstein SL, Ponseti IV. Curve progression in idiopathic scoliosis: long term follow-up. *J Bone Joint Surg [Am]* 1983;65A:447.

21. Weinstein SL, Zavala DC, Ponseti IV. Idiopathic scoliosis: long term follow-up. Prognosis in untreated patients. *J Bone Joint Surg [Am]* 1981;63A:702.

22. Wiltse LL. Spondylolisthesis: classification and etiology. Symposium on the Spine, American Academy of Orthopaedic Surgeons, 1969; pp. 143–166.

23. Winter RB. *Congenital spine deformity.* New York: Thieme Stratton; 1983.

24. Winter RB. Spinal problems in pediatric orthopaedics. In: Morrissy RT, ed. *Lovell and Winter's pediatric orthopaedics.* Philadelphia: JB Lippincott; 1990:697–698.

12

Case Histories

Questions and Answers

CASE HISTORY 1

What structure is most often compressed by herniation of the L4-5 disc?

1. L4 nerve root
2. L5 nerve root
3. S1 nerve root
4. L5 and S1 nerve roots
5. Cauda equina

Preferred response: 2

Discussion

The L5 nerve root is most often compressed by herniation of the L4-5 disc. However, the S1 nerve root can also be compressed by a posteromedial disc herniation at that level. An extreme lateral disc herniation can compress the nerve root exiting above the level of the herniation, in this case the L4 nerve root. Remember that a large central disc herniation can compress the lower sacral roots and cause bladder and bowel dysfunction (cauda equina syndrome).

References

1. Poss R, ed. Lumbar spine. In: *Orthopaedic knowledge update 3: home study syllabus.* Park Ridge, IL: American Academy of Orthopaedic Surgeons; 1990:459.
2. Wisneski RJ, Garfin SR, Rothman RH. Clinical syndrome of lumbar disc disease. In: Rothman RA, Simeone FA, eds. *The Spine.* 3rd ed. Philadelphia: WB Saunders; 1992:1:681–746.

CASE HISTORY 2

For 8 mo, a 59-yr-old man has had radiating upper extremity pain that extends from the neck down the lateral left arm and forearm and into the thumb and index finger. He complained of numbness over the tip of the thumb and dorsum of the left hand. On physical examination there was restricted motion of the cervical spine resulting from pain (especially in extension), weakness of the biceps muscle, and depression of the biceps reflex. There was no neurologic involvement in the lower extremities. Nonoperative treatment did not relieve his symptoms. An MRI scan (sagittal and axial) of the cervical spine is shown in Fig. 1A,B. The most appropriate treatment for this problem is:

1. Orthotic immobilization for 6 wk.
2. A neck extension exercise program.
3. Posterior decompressive laminectomy.

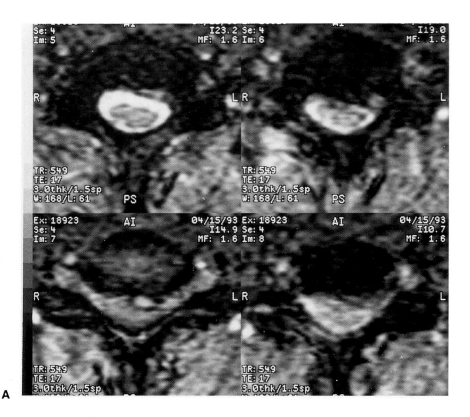

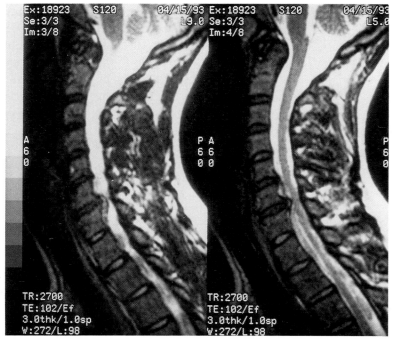

4. Anterior disc excision with fusion.
5. Posterior laminoplasty.

Preferred Response: 4

Discussion

The patient's symptoms were consistent with chronic disc degeneration and bony overgrowth with radiculopathy, had been persistent for 8 mo, and did not improve with conservative care. Posterior decompressive laminectomy alone would probably not be as beneficial as anterior approach with removal of any disc material or bony formation anterior to the nerve root. Likewise, laminoplasty would not address the anterior osteophyte deformation of the nerve root. Good results have been reported with anterior discectomy, removal of the offending bony bars, and anterior interbody fusion.

Reference

1. Herkowitz HN, Simeone FA, Blumberg KD, et al. Surgical management of cervical disc disease. In Rothman RH, Simeone FA, eds. *The spine.* 3rd ed. Philadelphia: WB Saunders, 1992;1:597–638.

CASE HISTORY 3

A 45-yr-old woman presented with complaints of low back pain radiating into her anterior left thigh. She stated that, although there was some gradual relief from the back pain, her leg pain continued. Physical examination revealed a positive femoral stretch sign on the right. An MRI scan of the lumbar spine (L3-4) is shown in Fig. 2. The most likely diagnosis is:

1. Spinal stenosis
2. Disc herniation
3. Facet syndrome
4. Conjoined root
5. Back strain

Preferred response: 2

Discussion

The MRI scan showed a foraminal disc herniation. This herniation can be easily missed by plain myelography because it may produce only a subtle medialization of the nerve root. The development of CT and MRI technology has made lateral herniations much easier to diagnose.

Reference

1. Bell GR, Modic MT. Radiology of the lumbar spine. In: Rothman RH, Simeone FA, eds. *The spine.* 3rd ed. Philadelphia: WB Saunders; 1992:1:125–153.

CASE HISTORY 4

What structure is at risk for possible injury if a right-sided surgical approach between C4-6 is used?

1. Superior laryngeal nerve
2. Recurrent laryngeal nerve
3. Internal laryngeal nerve
4. Thoracic duct
5. Esophagus

Preferred Response: 2

FIG. 1. A: Axial MRI of C5–6 level indicating bony overgrowth with posterior protrusion at this level. **B:** Sagittal MRI of the cervical spine demonstrating degenerative changes in the upper and middle part of the cervical spine and bony overgrowth and disc protrusion at C5–6.

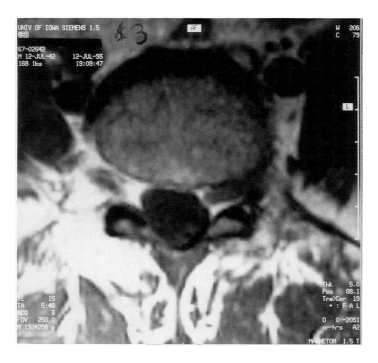

FIG. 2. Axial MRI scan of L3–4 disc level indicating left side foraminal disc herniation.

Discussion

The recurrent laryngeal nerve arises from the vagus nerve on the right side, at the level of the subclavian artery, and crosses from this to the tracheoesophageal groove. The laryngeal nerve is vulnerable to damage as it crosses at this level. Because its course in relation to the groove is more variable on the right than on the left, the nerve is more vulnerable to injury on the right side. The left recurrent laryngeal nerve branches out from the vagus nerve at the level of the arch of the aorta and subsequently ascends in the neck on the left side between the trachea and esophagus. Many right-handed surgeons prefer the approach to the right of the midline, and believe that orientation and technical performance is facilitated. Other surgeons believe that the side of the incision should be determined by the site of the predominant pathology.

Reference

1. Whitecloud TS III, Kelley LA. Anterior and posterior surgical approaches to the cervical spine. In: Frymoyer JW, ed. *The adult spine: principles and practice.* New York: Raven Press; 1991:2:991.

CASE HISTORY 5

The primary treatment regimen for a 33-yr-old man with acute-onset low back pain with no leg pain or other symptoms should include:

1. 1 to 2 days of bed rest
2. 1 to 2 wk of bed rest
3. Transcutaneous electrical nerve stimulation
4. Muscle relaxants
5. Traction

Preferred response: 1

Discussion

For the initial onset of low back pain, no more than 2 days of bed rest is recommended. Longer periods of inactivity result in deconditioning of the patient and do not improve pain. Transcutaneous nerve stimulation, muscle relaxants, and traction have not been demonstrated as effective in decreasing pain or muscle spasm.

References

1. Deyo RA, Diehl AK, Rosenthal M. How many days of bed rest for acute low back pain? A randomized clinical trial. *N Engl J Med* 1986;315:1064–1070.
2. Frymoyer JW, ed. Lumbar spine. In: *Orthopaedic knowledge update 4: home study syllabus.* Rosemont, IL: American Academy of Orthopaedic Surgeons; 1993:491–501.

CASE HISTORY 6

The most consistent finding in patients who have a cauda equina syndrome (CES) is:

1. Paralysis
2. Sensory deficits in the foot and ankle
3. Motor and sensory deficits distal to the knee
4. Fecal incontinence
5. Urinary retention

Preferred Response: 5

Discussion

Midline disc herniations occur in only about 1% to 2% of lumbar disc herniations. The most consistent finding is urinary retention. Patients with cauda equina syndrome typically do not feel that the bladder is distended (i.e. impaired afferent sacral nerve root function due to cauda equina compression). Other common findings are unilateral/bilateral sciatica, sensory and motor deficits, and abnormal straight leg raising. The most common sensory deficit occurs over the buttock, posterior-superior thighs, and peroneal regions (saddle anesthesia). Anal sphincter tone has been reported to be diminished in 60% to 80% of the cases.

Reference

1. Kostuik JP, Harrington I, Alexander D, et al. Cauda equina syndrome in lumbar disc herniation. *J Bone Joint Surg [Am]* 1986;68A:386–391.

CASE HISTORY 7

A 48-yr-old man injured his neck in a motor vehicle accident 4 wk prior to presentation. He complained of severe, nonradiating neck pain. Physical examination revealed restricted neck motion and no neurologic deficits. Anteroposterior and lateral radiographs revealed no abnormalities. The most appropriate diagnostic test would be:

1. MRI scan
2. CT scan/discography
3. Myelography
4. Flexion and extension lateral radiographs

5. Lateral tomograms

Preferred Response: 4

Discussion

Ligamentous and soft-tissue injuries may go unrecognized. Physician-supervised flexion-extension radiographs are indicated in the presence of persistent pain following trauma. Differences in angular deformity greater than 11 degrees between adjacent vertebrae or translational displacement greater than 3.5 mm indicates the presence of instability from a soft tissue injury.

References

1. Dunn EJ, Blazar S. Soft tissue injuries of the lower cervical spine. In Griffin PP, ed. *American Academy of Orthopaedic Surgeons Instructional Course Lectures,* XXXVII. Park Ridge, IL: American Academy of Orthopaedic Surgeons; 1987:499–512.
2. White AA III, Johnson RM, Panjabi MM, et al. Biomechanical analysis of clinical stability of the cervical spine. *Clin Orthop* 1975;109:85–96.

CASE HISTORY 8

After vigorous activity, a 48-yr-old man experienced pain in his right leg. He sought medical attention and was initially treated with rest and nonsteroidal anti-inflammatory agents. A CT scan of the lumbar spine was performed. His symptoms did not hinder his ability to work, but he had continued minimal low back pain and mild lower extremity pain after vigorous sports activity. Neurologic examination was normal, with a straight leg raising test equivocal at 80 degrees. Recommended treatment should be:

1. Percutaneous discectomy
2. Open surgical disc excision
3. Lumbar spine fusion
4. Continued nonsurgical care
5. Chemonucleolysis

Preferred Response: 4

Discussion

This patient had a herniated lumbar disc, but his symptoms abated and he returned to full function. Because the indications for lumbar disc surgery are incapacitating leg pain (sciatic) combined with positive nerve root tension signs (straight leg raising, SLR test, or Lasegue's test) invasive treatment is not indicated despite abnormal findings on CT scan.

References

1. Garfin SR, Rydevik BL, Brown RA: Compression neuropathy of spinal nerve roots: a mechanical or biological problem? *Spine* 1991;16:162–166.
2. Weber H. Lumbar disc herniation: a controlled, prospective study with ten years of observation. *Spine* 1983;8:131–140.

CASE HISTORY 9

What is the occurrence of abnormality on MRI scan of the cervical spine in asymptomatic subjects over the age of 40?

1. 81% to 100%
2. 61% to 80%
3. 41% to 60%
4. 21% to 40%
5. 0% to 20%

Preferred Response: 4

Discussion

As demonstrated in a recently published prospective study, 28% of asymptomatic subjects over the age of 40 have evidence of a herniated disc or foraminal stenosis on MRI examination. This high prevalence of abnormal cervical MRIs in asymptomatic people emphasizes the need to correlate radiographic findings with clinical symptoms and examinations.

Reference

1. Boden SD, McCown PR, David DO, et al. Abnormal magnetic resonance scan of the cervical spine in asymptomatic subjects: a prospective investigation. *J Bone Joint Surg [Am]* 1990;72A:1178–1184.

CASE HISTORY 10

Among normal subjects under the age of 40, what is the likelihood that anatomic evidence of a herniated disc of the lumbar spine will be found by imaging techniques such as myelography, CT, or MRI?

1. 10% to 15%
2. 21% to 30%
3. 31% to 40%
4. 41% to 50%
5. Greater than 50%

Preferred Response: 2

Discussion

Radiologic evidence of lumbar disc herniation is found in 20% to 30% of normal people. In these instances, herniations are asymptomatic and result in no clinical disease.

References

1. Boden SD, David DO, Dina TS, et al. Abnormal magnetic resonance scans of the lumbar spine in asymptomatic subjects: a prospective investigation. *J Bone Joint Surg [Am]* 1990; 72A:403–408.
2. Wiesel SW, Tsourmas N, Feffer HL, et al. A study of computer assisted tomography. I: The incidence of positive CAT scan in an asymptomatic group of patients. *Spine* 1984;9:549–551.

CASE HISTORY 11

A 40-yr-old woman presented with complaints of neck pain radiating to the dorsum of her right hand and extending to her middle finger and the radial aspect of her ring finger. She also had weakness of the right wrist flexors, pronation of the right forearm, and a mild decrease in the triceps reflex of the right arm. Biceps and brachioradialis reflexes were normal. The most likely diagnosis is:

1. Herniated disc at C4-5
2. Herniated disc at C5-6
3. Herniated disc at C6-7
4. Syrinx of the cervical spinal cord
5. Intramedullary spinal cord tumor at C-5

Preferred Response: 3

Discussion

The patient's sensory and motor deficits are consistent with a right C7 radiculopathy from a herniated disc at C6-7.

References

1. Hoppenfeld S. *Orthopaedic neurology: a diagnostic guide to neurologic levels.* Philadelphia: JB Lippincott; 1977.

2. Simeone FA. Cervical disc disease with radiculopathy. In: Rothman RH, Simeone FA, eds. *The spine.* 3rd ed. Philadelphia: WB Saunders, 1992;1:553–560.

CASE HISTORY 12

The most sensitive test for the early diagnosis of discitis is:

1. CT scan
2. MRI scan
3. Gallium scan
4. Technetium bone scan
5. Plain radiograph

Preferred Response: 2

Discussion

Diagnosis of infection of the intervertebral disc is often delayed by the normal results demonstrated on plain radiographs. In the past, the most useful technique was radionuclide imaging. However, technetium and gallium scans rely on the infection producing an increased blood supply to the area as a result of acute inflammation. In the early stages when the infection is confined to the relatively avascular disc space, these scans may be of little value. In addition, radionuclide imaging involves the use of ionizing radiation, and in the case of gallium imaging, definitive results are not obtained for 24 to 48 hr, with a significant number of false positive results. MRI scan has been shown to be a very sensitive test for discitis with the findings of decreased signal from the affected disc on T1-weighted images and an increased signal on T2 images. The CT scan can show destructive lesions before plain radiographs, but destruction must occur before positive findings are seen.

References

1. Modic MT, Feiglin DH, Piraino DW, et al. Vertebral osteomyelitis: assessment using MR. *Radiology* 1985;157:157–166.
2. Szypryt EP, Hardy JG, Hinton CE, et al. A comparison between magnetic resonance imaging and scintigraphic bone imaging in the diagnosis of disc space infection in an animal model. *Spine* 1988;13:1042–1048.

CASE HISTORY 13

A 55-yr-old woman had a 12 yr progressive history of low back pain radiating to her thighs bilaterally. She had undergone a L4-S1 posterior fusion 15 yr ago. Radiographs show 7 mm of displacement of L-3 on L-4 in flexion as compared to in extension. Based on these clinical and radiographic findings, the most likely diagnosis is:

1. Pseudoarthrosis
2. Isthmic spondylolisthesis
3. Vertebral metastatic destruction
4. L3-4 "instability"
5. L4-S1 spinal stenosis

Preferred Response: 4

Discussion

After lumbar fusion, adjacent segments are at risk for the later development of a variety of degenerative changes that may be either asymptomatic or symptomatic and may include clinical and radiographic features of degenerative spinal stenosis, segmental instability, or lumbar disc herniation. The dominant reason for these degenerative changes is mechanical. Inadvertent damage of the facets or facet denervation may be contributory.

References

1. Lehmann TR, Spratt KF, Tozzi JE, et al. Long-term followup of lower lumbar fusion patients. *Spine* 1987;12:97–104.
2. Stokes IA, Wilder DG, Frymoyer JW, et al. Assessment of patients with low back pain by biplanar radiographic measurement of the intervertebral motion. *Spine* 1981;6:233–240.

CASE HISTORY 14

A 48-yr-old woman presented with severe L5 radiculopathy caused by a herniated disc at L4-5. A CT scan confirmed the diagnosis, and surgical disc excision was performed. Lower extremity pain was relieved by the surgery, but the moderate low back pain persisted. The long-term (10-yr) prognosis is:

1. Continued moderate low back pain
2. Progressive, severe low back pain
3. Gradual resolution of low back pain
4. Recurrent lower extremity symptoms
5. Spinal instability

Preferred Response: 3

Discussion

Severe radicular pain that does not resolve with nonsurgical measures is the primary indication for surgical disc excision. With a proper diagnosis and meticulous surgical technique, relief of radicular symptoms can be expected in about 90% of patients. Ten percent to 15% of patients will have back pain after the surgery. Long-term studies show that the pain will gradually diminish with time. Recurrently, radiculopathy after surgery occurs in only 5% to 7% of patients.

References

1. Hakelius A. Prognosis in sciatica: a clinical followup of surgical and nonsurgical treatment. *Acta Orthop Scand [Suppl]* 1970;129:1–76.
2. Hanley EN, Shapiro DE. The development of low back pain after excision of a lumbar disc. *J Bone Joint Surg [Am]* 1989;71A:719–721.
3. Weber H. Lumbar disc herniation: a controlled, prospective study with ten years of observation. *Spine* 1983;8:131–140.

CASE HISTORY 15

The prevalence of disc degeneration and/or bulging of a lumbar disc at one or more levels in patients over age 60 yr is:

1. 0% to 10%
2. 11% to 25%
3. 26% to 50%
4. 51% to 75%
5. 76% to 100%

Preferred Response: 5

Discussion

In a recently published prospective study, degenerated or bulging discs were identified in 93% of asymptomatic subjects over the age of 60. The same abnormalities were identified in 35% of subjects younger than age 40. Clinical symptoms and findings, however, must correlate with abnormal radiographic studies to make appropriate therapeutic recommendations.

Reference

1. Boden SD, David DO, Dina TS, et al. Abnormal magnetic resonance scans of the lumbar spine in asymptomatic subjects: a prospective investigation. *J Bone Joint Surg [Am]* 1990; 72A:403–408.

CASE HISTORY 16

In a primary care setting, approximately 4% of patients who present with back pain will have spinal compression fractures and 3% will have spondylolisthesis. What percentage are thought to have a spinal neoplasm (primary or metastatic)?

1. Less than 1%
2. 5%
3. 10%
4. 20%
5. 25%

Preferred Response: 1

Discussion

Only about 0.7% of patients with back pain seen in a primary care setting are proven to have a malignant primary or metastatic spine neoplasm. Even fewer have ankylosing spondylitis (about 0.3%) or spinal infection (0.1%).

References

1. Deyo RA, Diehl AK. Cancer as a cause of back pain: frequency, clinical presentation, and diagnostic strategies. *J Gen Intern Med* 1988;3; 230–238.
2. Liang M, Komaroff AL. Roentgenograms in primary care patients with acute back pain: a cost effectiveness analysis. *Arch Intern Med* 1982;142:1108–1112.

CASE HISTORY 17

The most common complications from anterior cervical fusion surgery for a herniated disc occur as a result of:

1. The type of surgical approach to the cervical spine.

2. Excision of the herniated disc.
3. Harvesting of bone graft from the iliac crest.
4. Placement of bone graft between adjacent vertebrae.
5. Failure to drain the cervical incision.

Preferred Response: 3

Discussion

The highest frequency of complications occurs at the iliac donor site (approximately 20%). Included are hematoma, superficial and deep infection, and lateral femoral cutaneous nerve neurapraxia. The incidence of surgical site problems is much smaller.

Reference

1. Gore DR, Sepic SB. Anterior cervical fusion for degenerated or protruded discs: a review of one hundred forty-six patients. *Spine* 1984;9:667–671.

CASE HISTORY 18

The bulbocavernosus reflex can be permanently interrupted with injuries to what spinal anatomic region?

1. Brain
2. Cervical spine
3. Thoracic spine
4. Thoracolumbar spine
5. Sciatic nerve

Preferred Response: 4

Discussion

The injury most likely to cause disruption of the bulbocavernosus reflex is one that affects the conus medullaris (located at the thoracolumbar junction).

Reference

1. Keenan TL, Benson DR. Initial evaluation of the spine: injured patient. In: Browner BD, Jupiter JB, Levine AM, et al. (eds): *Skeletal trauma.* Philadelphia: WB Saunders; 1992.

CASE HISTORY 19

A 40-yr-old barber presented with a 10-wk history of low back and leg pain. An MRI scan (sagittal and axial) is shown in Fig. 3A,B. The most specific physical finding to verify the clinical significance of this patient's condition is:

1. Loss of sensation
2. Muscle weakness
3. A positive ipsilateral straight leg raising test
4. A positive contralateral straight leg raising test
5. Diminished reflex

Preferred Response: 4

Discussion

Positive contralateral straight leg raising test is the most specific finding indicative of neural irritability. The pain must radiate past the knee on the symptomatic side when the opposite leg is raised. However, a positive ipsilateral straight leg raising test with pain radiating below the knee is also of diagnostic value. The presence of back or thigh pain is not considered a specific diagnostic sign.

References

1. Lumbar spine. In Frymoyer JW, ed. *Orthopaedic knowledge update 4: home study syllabus.* Rosemont, IL: American Academy of Orthopaedic Surgeons; 1993:491–501.
2. Spangfort EV. The lumbar disc herniation: a computer-aided analysis of 2504 operations. *Acta Orthop Scand* 1972;142(suppl):1–95.
3. Waddell G, McCulloch JA, Kummel E, et al. Non-organic physical signs in low back pain. *Spine* 1980;5:117–125.

CASE HISTORY 20

In frequency as a reason for office visits to a physician, back pain ranks:

1. First
2. Second
3. Third
4. Fourth
5. Fifth

Preferred Response: 2

Discussion

Back pain ranks second only to upper respiratory tract illness as a symptomatic reason for office visits to physicians. About 70% of adults have low back pain at some time, but only 14% have an episode that lasts more than 2 wk. About 1.5% of such episodes have features of sciatica.

References

1. Cypress BK. Characteristics of physician visits for back symptoms: a national perspective. *Am J Public Health* 1983;73:389–395.
2. Deyo RA, Loeser JD, Bigos JS. Herniated lumbar intervertebral disc. *Ann Intern Med* 1990;112:598–603.
3. Deyo RA, Tsui-Wu YJ. Descriptive epidemiology of low back pain and its related medical care in the United States. *Spine* 1987;12:264–268.

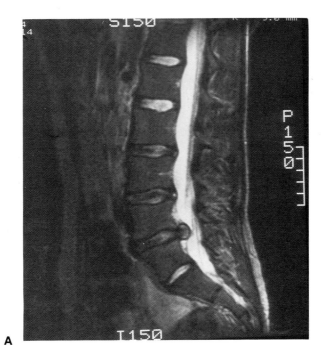

A

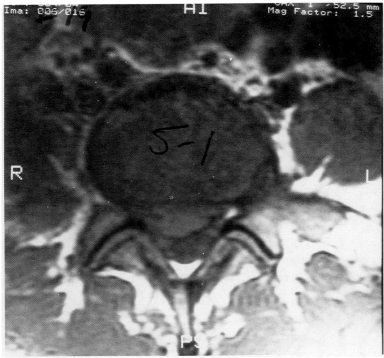

B

FIG. 3. Sagittal and axial MRI scans of the lumbar spine indicating disc herniation at the L5–S1 level.

CASE HISTORY 21

A 36-yr-old woman presents with a 6-mo history of progressive bilateral leg weakness and a spastic gait. Examination reveals hyperreflexia, bilateral upgoing toes (positive Babinski), and 4/5 proximal right and left leg weakness. Sensory level is just above the umbilicus. MRI is seen in Fig. 4A,B. The most likely diagnosis is:

1. Intradural extramedullary meningioma/neurofibroma
2. Thoracic disc herniation
3. Thoracic spinal stenosis
4. Thoracic spinal fracture

Preferred Response: 2

Discussion

The patient has a progressive thoracic myelopathy. The onset of a fracture would be sudden. Thoracic spinal stenosis is extremely rare. Intradural extramedullary tumors tend to be, but are not necessarily, asymmetric (usually posterolateral). A midline thoracic disc herniation presents primarily with a symmetric myelopathy and mild or no radiculopathy. Because the condition is limited to the midline, treatment is a transthoracic disc removal.

References

1. Arce CA, Dohrmann GJ. Herniated thoracic disks. *Neurol Clin* 1985;3:383–392.
2. Dietze DD Jr, Fessler RG. Thoracic disc herniation. *Neurosurg Clin North Am* 1993; 4:75–89.
3. Sekhar LN, Jannetta PJ. Thoracic disc herniation: operative approaches and results. *Neurosurgery* 1983;12:303–305.

CASE HISTORY 22

A 45-yr-old man presents with a 3-mo history of right arm pain and weakness with no history of trauma. Curtailing his usual activities as well as wearing a soft collar and taking anti-inflammatory medicines did not significantly affect his symptoms. Examination revealed an absent right triceps reflex, a weak right triceps muscle (3/5), and decreased sensation on the palmar surface of the right index finger. The most likely diagnosis is:

1. Neck strain
2. C5-6 disc herniation
3. C6-7 disc herniation
4. Neurogenic thoracic outlet syndrome
5. Carpal tunnel syndrome

Preferred Response: 3

Discussion

This is a clear case of C7 radiculopathy caused by a soft C6-7 disc herniation on the right (Fig. 5A,B). The C7 root innervates the triceps muscle, contributes to the triceps reflex, and clinically controls sensation of the index and long fingers. A neck strain does not usually present with arm symptoms. A C6 radiculopathy associated with a C5-6 disc herniation would present with biceps muscle weakness, a decreased biceps reflex and decreased sensation in the thumb. Neurogenic thoracic outlet syndrome presents clinically with atrophy of the intrinsic muscles of the hand and more of an inferior brachial plexus involvement, specifically more C8 problems. Carpal tunnel syndrome is not asso-

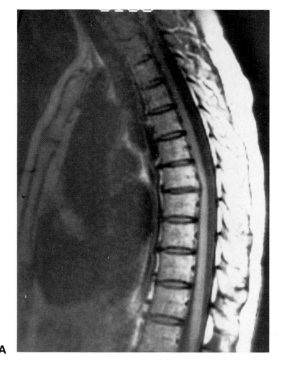

A

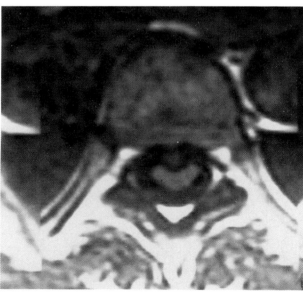

B

FIG. 4. A: Sagittal magnetic resonance image of the thoracic spine demonstrating anterior indentation at T7-8 concomitant with a thoracic disc herniation. **B:** Axial magnetic resonance image of the thoracic spine showing the midline anterior thoracic herniated disc herniation at T7-8 compressing the spinal cord.

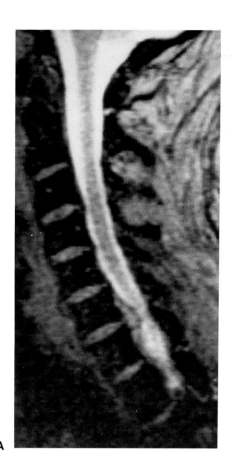

A

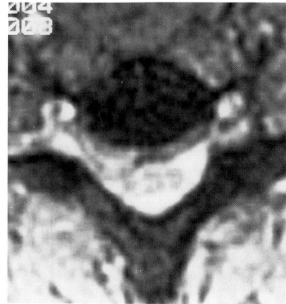

B

FIG. 5. Axial **(A)** and **(B)** sagittal T2-weighted magnetic resonance image of the cervical spine. A large free fragment of disc is demonstrated at C6-7 deforming the spinal cord. On the axial cut, obliteration of the subarachnoid space and nerve root on the right is also seen.

ciated with triceps weakness, or triceps reflex changes, and the loss of sensation would be seen in the thumb, index, and long finger.

References

1. Campbell AM, Phillips DG. Cervical disc lesion with neurological disorder: differential diagnosis, treatment and prognosis. *Br Med J* 1960;5197:481–485.
2. Dillin W, Booth R, Cuckler J, et al. Cervical radiculopathy: a review. *Spine* 1986;11: 988–991.
3. Lipson SJ. Cervical disc disease: pathogenesis and natural history. *Sem Spine Surg* 1989;1:190–193.

CASE HISTORY 23

A 29-yr-old man had a 6-mo history of sudden onset of back pain and left leg pain radiating to the lateral aspect of the left foot. The pain was aggravated by ambulation and improved with rest. There was no history of trauma. The patient had no problems with bowel or bladder control. Examination revealed a positive straight leg raising test to 60° on the left and an absent left Achilles reflex. MR imaging of the lower lumbar spine is seen in Fig. 6A,B. The most likely diagnosis is:

1. Synovial cyst of the lumbar area
2. Neurofibroma of the cauda equina
3. Herniated lumbar disc at left L5-S1
4. Herniated lumbar disc at left L4-L5

Preferred Response: 3

Discussion

The patient's history and physical examination were classic for an S1

radiculopathy caused by a herniated disc at L5-S1 on the left. The pattern of pain was in the S1 distribution rather than L5, which would primarily radiate to the large toe not the lateral part of the foot. The Achilles reflex is also innervated primarily by S1. Neurofibroma of the cauda equina clinically presents with pain that does not improve with rest. In fact, with an intrathecal mass such as an neurofibroma, the pain is often made worse when the patient rests. Synovial cysts of the lumbar spine are rare and the onset of the pain is seldom sudden.

References

1. Frymoyer JW. Back pain and sciatica. *N Engl J Med* 1988;318:291–300.
2. Liu SS, Williams KD, Drayer BP, Spetzler RF, Sonntag VKH. Synovial cysts of the lumbosacral spine: diagnosis by MR imaging. *AJNR* 1989;10:1239–1242.
3. Pappas CTE, Harrington T, Sonntag VKH. Outcome analysis in 654 surgically treated lumbar disc herniations. *Neurosurgery* 1992;30: 862–866.

CASE HISTORY 24

A 75-yr-old man presented with a 2-yr history of low back pain and bilateral leg pain made worse by standing and walking. The patient related that he could walk only one to two blocks before his leg began feeling heavy with increasing pain. He then had to stop and rest several minutes before he could walk again. He had no history of urinary incontinence or impotence. He had, however, experienced a recent onset of urgency and frequency of urination. Examination revealed decreased reflexes in the legs with no associated motor or sensory

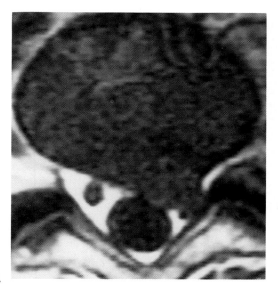

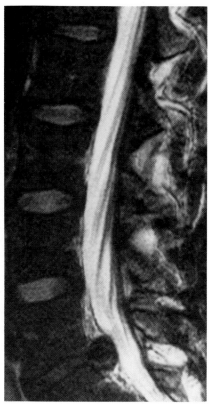

A **B**

FIG. 6. A: Axial magnetic resonance image showing a left HNP at L5-S1. **B:** Sagittal magnetic resonance image demonstrating a large L5-S1 HNP.

deficit. Straight leg raising test, "fabere" sign (flexion, abduction, external rotation, extension of the hip), and the dorsalis pedis pulses are normal. Lateral myelogram and axial CT scans are seen in Fig. 7A and B. The most likely diagnosis is:

1. Vascular insufficiency of the lower extremities
2. Lumbar spinal stenosis
3. Metastatic epidural tumor
4. Bilateral hip disease

Preferred Response: 2

Discussion

This is a classic presentation of lumbar stenosis that presents with leg symptoms exacerbated by walking and a normal physical examination. The major differential diagnosis is vascular insufficiency (Leriche's syndrome); however, this patient has normal pulses in his feet and no pain whatsoever at rest. Metastatic tumor has a shorter history and symptoms should be present at rest as well. Hip disease rarely presents bilaterally and should have a positive "fabere" sign.

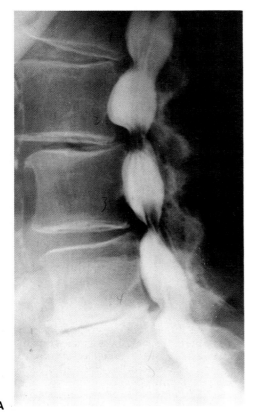
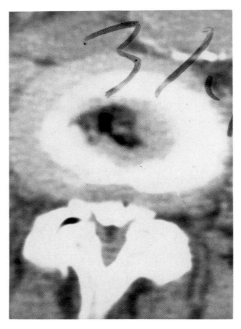

A   **B**

FIG. 7. A: Lateral lumbar myelogram showing severe stenosis at L2-3, L3-4, and moderate stenosis at L1-2 and L4-5. **B:** Axial postmyelogram computed tomography with severe stenosis secondary to hypertrophied facets and ligament flavum at L3-4.

References

1. Kirkaldy-Willis WH, Wedge JH, Yong-Hing K, et al. Pathology and pathogenesis of lumbar spondylosis and stenosis. *Spine* 1978;3: 319–328.
2. Schönström NSR, Bolender N-F, Spengler DM. The pathomorphology of spinal stenosis as seen on CT scans of the lumbar spine. *Spine* 1985;10(9):806–811.
3. Wilson CB. Significance of the small lumbar spinal canal: cauda equina compression syndromes due to spondylosis. Part 3: intermittent claudication. *J Neurosurg* 1969;31:499–506.

CASE HISTORY 25

This 64-yr-old woman had a 2-yr history of bilateral arm weakness and intermittent pain in the lateral parts of both arms, the right greater than left. During the last 6 mo, she also experienced difficulty with gait and frequency of urination. Examination revealed 4/5 weakness of both upper extremities, proximally more than distally, and bilateral weakness of the iliopsoas (4/5) and quadriceps (3/5) weakness.

She had absent biceps reflexes but increased triceps, patellar, and Achilles reflexes and bilateral upgoing toes. Sensation was grossly normal except decreased vibration sense in the legs. MRI is seen in Fig. 8. The most likely diagnosis is:

1. Intramedullary cervical cord tumor
2. Cervical spinal stenosis
3. Nerve sheath tumor of the upper cervical spine
4. Syringomyelia of the cervical cord

Preferred Response: 2

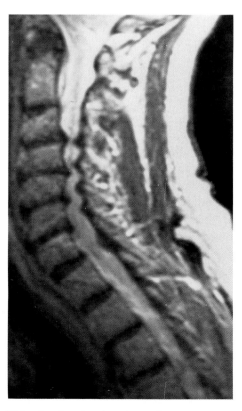

FIG. 8. Sagittal magnetic resonance image (T2-weighted) of the cervical spine showing severe cervical spinal stenosis from C3 to C6.

Discussion

The patient has a clinical picture of a cervical myeloradiculopathy secondary to cervical spinal stenosis. Intramedullary cord tumor and syringomyelia present clinically with a sensory disassociation; dorsal column intact but impairment of the spinothalamic tract usually presenting with a cape-like sensory deficit over the shoulder. Also, pain is an atypical presentation of the latter two. Nerve sheath tumor can present with a myelopathy but the radicular component is usually limited to one particular nerve root and is not bilateral.

References

1. Herkowitz HN. A comparison of anterior cervical fusion, cervical laminectomy, and cervical laminoplasty for the surgical management of multiple level spondylotic radiculopathy. *Spine* 1988;13:774–780.
2. Hoff JT, Wilson CB. The pathophysiology of cervical spondylotic radiculopathy and myelopathy. *Clin Neurosurg* 1977;24:474–487.
3. Raynor RB. Anterior or posterior approach to the cervical spine: an anatomical and radiographic evaluation and comparison. *Neurosurgery* 1983;146:27–28.

CASE HISTORY 26

A 12-yr-old girl who is premenarchal presents with a 30° right thoracic scoliosis T5-12, apex T-8. Neurologic exam is normal. Her Risser grade is I. You would recommend to the family.

1. Observation (return 4 mo)
2. Posterior spinal fusion and instrumentation
3. Electrical stimulation

4. Anterior and posterior spinal fusion with posterior instrumentation
5. TLSO

Preferred Response: 5

Discussion

The patient should be treated with a spinal orthosis. TLSOs are most commonly used, yet the Milwaukee brace remains the "gold standard." The indication is based on the 90% probability of curve progression in this skeletally immature, premenarchal patient. Surgery is only indicated here for progression despite bracing. Electrical stimulation has been tried in the past but was a failure. Anterior fusion to supplant posterior fusion is only indicated in patients <10 yr old requiring spinal fusion (Table 1).

References

1. Lonstein JE, Carlson JM. The prediction of curve progression in untreated idiopathic scoliosis during growth. *J Bone Joint Surg [Am]* 1984;66:1061–1071.
2. Nachemson A, Lonstein J, Weinsten S (1982). Report of the SRS Prevalence and Natural History Committee 1982. Presented at SRS meeting, Denver.

TABLE 1. *Probability of progression: magnitude of curve at initial detection versus age*

Curve magnitude at detection (degrees)	Age at detection (yr)		
	10–12	13–15	16
<19	25%	10%	0%
20–29	60	40	10
30–59	90	70	30
>60	100	90	70

CASE HISTORY 27

An 8-day-old infant is sent to you because of a pelvic obliquity. Neurologic exam is normal. The labor and delivery history is unremarkable. This is the first child in the family. AP radiographs are seen in Fig. 9. You would recommend:

1. CT scan of LS area
2. Renal ultrasound
3. EKG
4. MRI of spinal cord
5. Polytomography of LS spine

Preferred Response: 2

Discussion

Twenty percent to 40% of patients with congenital spinal abnormalities have an associated genitourinary tract abnormality. Six percent of these are potentially life threatening. Renal ultrasound is the screening test of choice. IVP and retrograde urograms may be necessary to study lower tracts. The most common findings are unilateral kidney, duplication of the kidney, and ureteric obstruction.

References

1. Drvac DJ, Ruderman RJ, Coonrad RW, et al. Congenital scoliosis and urinary tract abnormalities. *J Pediatr Orthop* 1987;7: 441–443.
2. MacEwen GD, Winter RB, Hardy JH. Evaluation of kidney anomalies in congenital scoliosis. *J Bone Joint Surg [Am]* 1972;6454: 1341–1454.

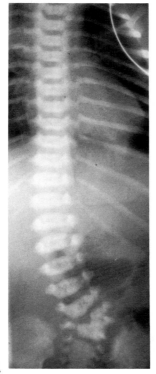 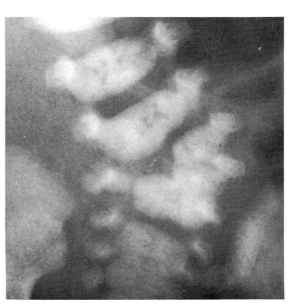

A   B

FIG. 9. A: Eight-day-old infant with 2 lumbosacral hemivertebrae. Because of the curve progression he was indicated for hemivertebrae resection. **B:** Spot AP radiograph demonstrating 2 hemivertebrae. (Case courtesy of Stuart L. Weinstein, M.D., University of Iowa.)

CASE HISTORY 28

Treatment indications for lumbar hemivertebrae in the future will most likely be:

1. Observation only
2. Posterior spinal fusion
3. Anterior and posterior spinal fusion
4. Hemivertebrectomy and fusion
5. Orthotics

Preferred Response: 4

Discussion

The lumbosacral hemivertebrae is the one generally agreed upon indication for hemivertebrectomy and fusion. Congenital curves are not braceable and progression is almost a certainty in this case with a supra-pelvic cause of permanent obliquity unless treated.

References

1. Bradford DS, Boachie-Adjei O. One-stage anterior and posterior hemivertebral resection and

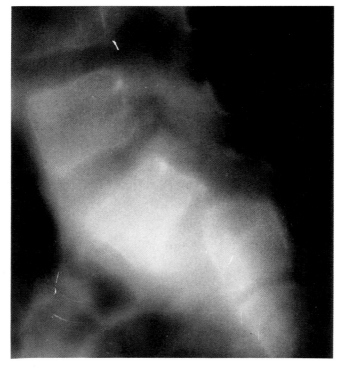

FIG. 10

arthrodesis. *J Bone Joint Surg [Am]* 1990;72:
536–540.
2. Weinstein SL. *Pediatric spine: principles and
practice.* New York: Raven Press; 1994.

CASE HISTORY 29

A 9-yr-old girl presents to you with a
gait abnormality. She has a short stride
length and walks with her legs externally
rotated. She denies back pain. Passively
her legs can be elevated more than six
inches off the exam table before she
begins to "rock" her plevis. On forward
flexion she has a palpable step-off at L5-
S1 (Fig. 10). Treatment would include:

1. S1 nerve root decompression
2. L5-S1 posterolateral fusion
3. L4-S1 posterolateral fusion
4. L-5 vertebrectomy
5. L-5 laminectomy

Preferred Response: 3

Discussion

This patient presents with a Type 1
spondylolisthesis. She has a significant
kyphotic deformity at the lumbosacral
junction. Even though she has no pain her
spondylolisthesis is manifest by a severe
gait disturbance and tight hamstrings. In
children an L-4 to sacrum posterolateral
fusion is the treatment recommended. This
would usually be accompanied by reduc-

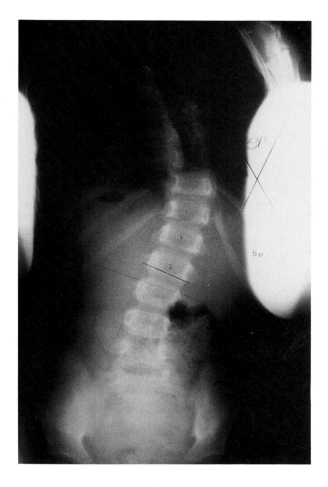

FIG. 11

tion and casting. Vertebrectomy, nerve root decompression are not necessary. Laminectomy alone is contraindicated; it must always be accompanied by a fusion and an L5-sacrum fusion would be inadequate to prevent further slippage.

References

1. Brunet JA, Wiley JJ. Acquired spondylolysis after spinal fusion. *J Bone Joint Surg [Br]* 1984;66B:720–724.
2. Weinstein SL. *Pediatric spine: principles and practice*. New York: Raven Press; 1994.

CASE HISTORY 30

A 5-yr-old boy presents to you with a 55° right thoracic scoliosis seen in Fig. 11. He is neurologically normal. He is the product of a normal labor and delivery. Parents thought the spine was normal one yr ago. You would recommend:

1. MRI of the brain and spinal cord
2. Renal ultrasound
3. Anterior spine fusion and posterior spine fusion

4. Posterior spine fusion
5. Orthotic treatment

Preferred Response: 1

Discussion

This patient presents at an early age an unusually long curve with minimal pedicle rotation. MRI is indicated in unusual curve patterns (e.g. left thoracic curves), early onset scoliosis (less than 10 yr of age), rapidly progressive curves, patients with any neurologic deficiency, or patients with persistent pain of uncertain etiology.

This patient had a halocord syrinx and a Chiari malformation. His scoliosis resolved after neurosurgical treatment of his brain and spinal cord lesions.

References

1. Hugus JJ, Taylor TFK, McGee-Collett M, Besser M, Gurr KR. Syringomyelia and scoliosis: a new view. Presented at the 25th annual meeting of the Scoliosis Research Society, Honolulu, Hawaii, September 27, 1990.
2. Muhonen MG, Menezes AH, Sawin PD, Weinstein SL. Scoliosis in pediatric Chiari malformations without myelodysplasia. *J Neurosurg* 1992;77:69–77.

Subject Index